Turning an old Mattress into fresh Marijuana

Copyright

Marijuana
Growing Guide

Here is some foam in a box where we can make any atmospheric condition, any temperature, and any weather. The local farmers have taught us so much about how to grow things hydroponically.

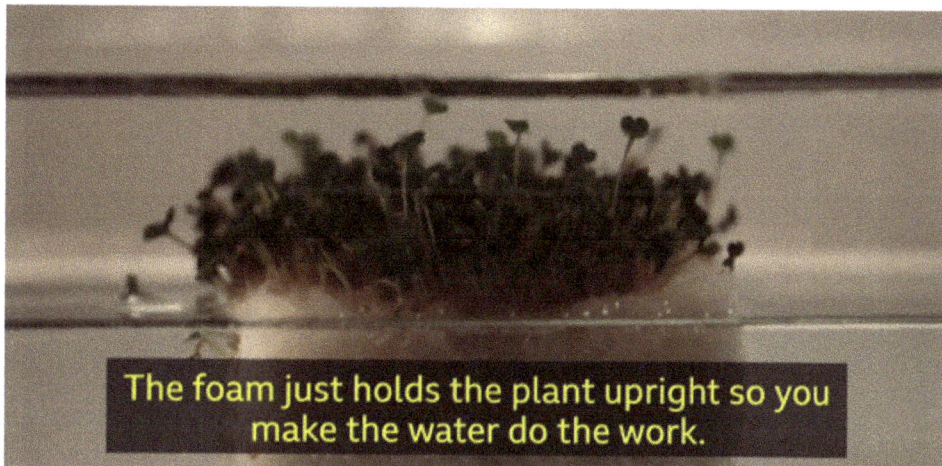

The foam just holds the plant upright so you make the water do the work.

The foam just holds the plant upright so you make the water do the work. All the other functions of the soil come from the nutrients in the water. You can use 20% of the water that you would take to grow something in the ground.

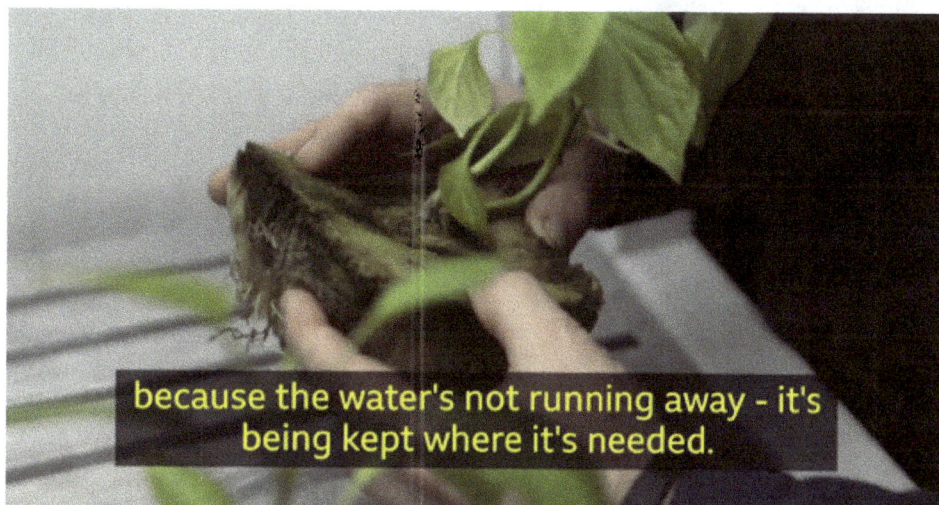

because the water's not running away - it's being kept where it's needed.

Because the water is not running away. It is being kept where it is needed.

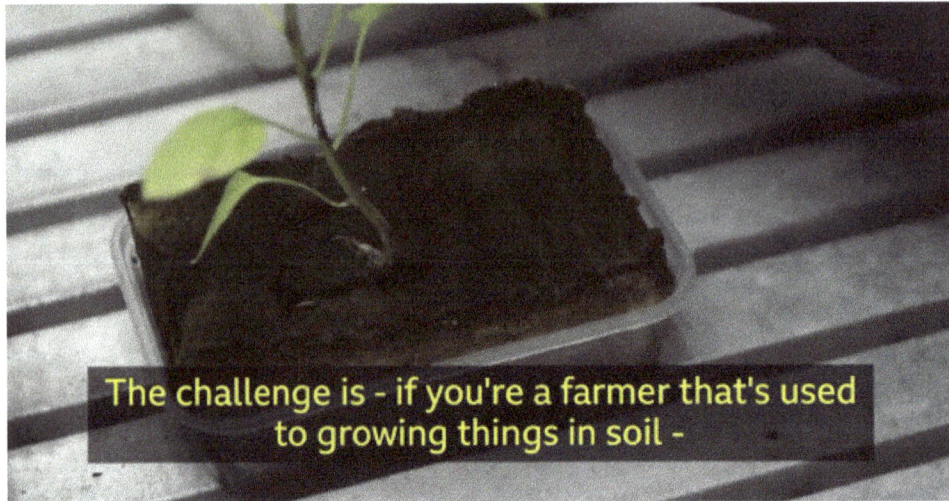

The challenge is - if you're a farmer that's used to growing things in soil -

The Challenge is – if you are a farmer that is used to growing things in soil - being asked to grow things in foam's a big ask.

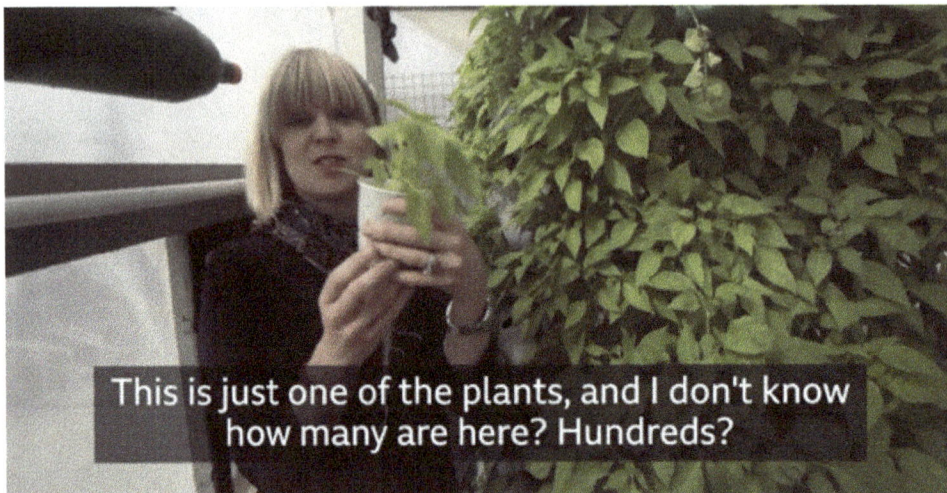

This is just one of the plants, and I don't know how many are here? Hundreds?

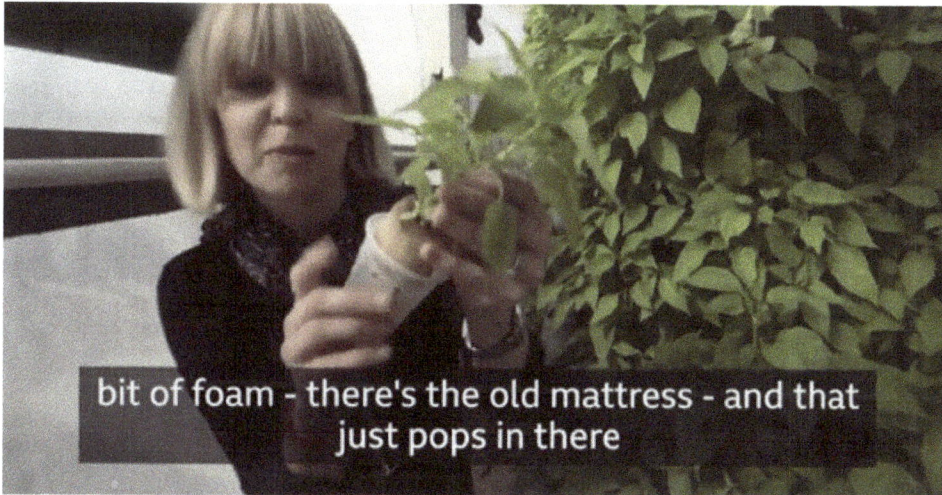

bit of foam - there's the old mattress - and that just pops in there

With a coffee cup, and a bit of foam, you can grow any plant.

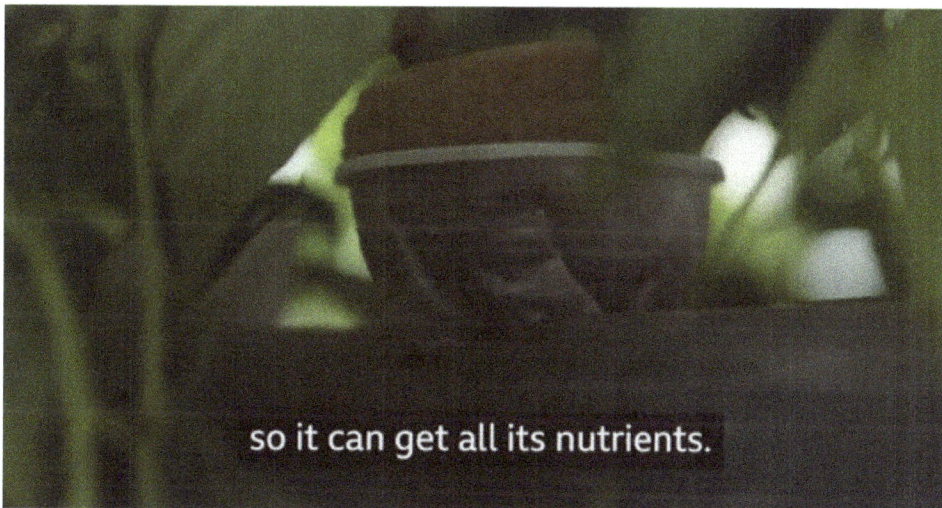

so it can get all its nutrients.

Just place the cup in the water so the plant can get all its nutrients.

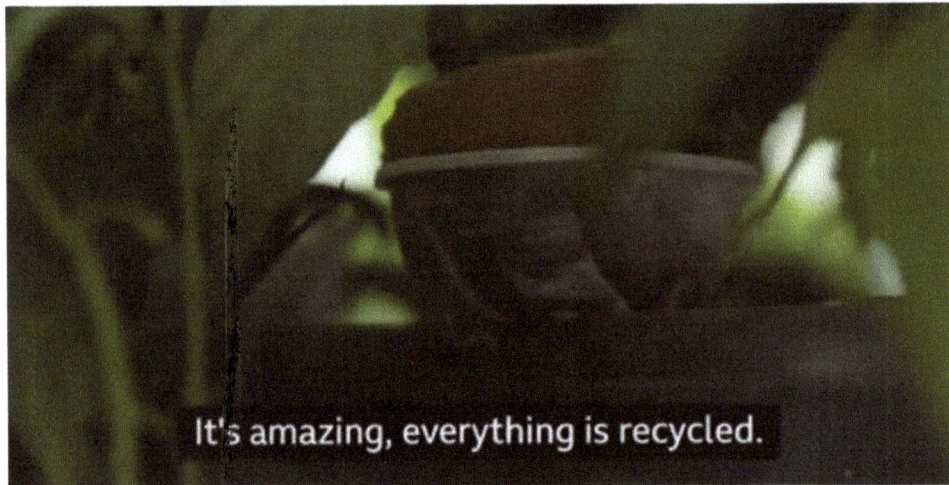

It's amazing, everything is recycled.

This is truly amazing, everything is recycled, and you make money too. Thousands of people have learnt this technique, and they are making money.

Using an old mattresses to grow plants is fantastic. It is a great step for urban agriculture around the world. There is a lot that anybody that lives in an urban environment, can learn from this book. It is all about taking value from things that can be re-used and recycled and making the absolute most out of a very limited space and really limited resources. And as urban environments face a changing climate and those limited resources in the future, that is a reality that we are all going to have to face.

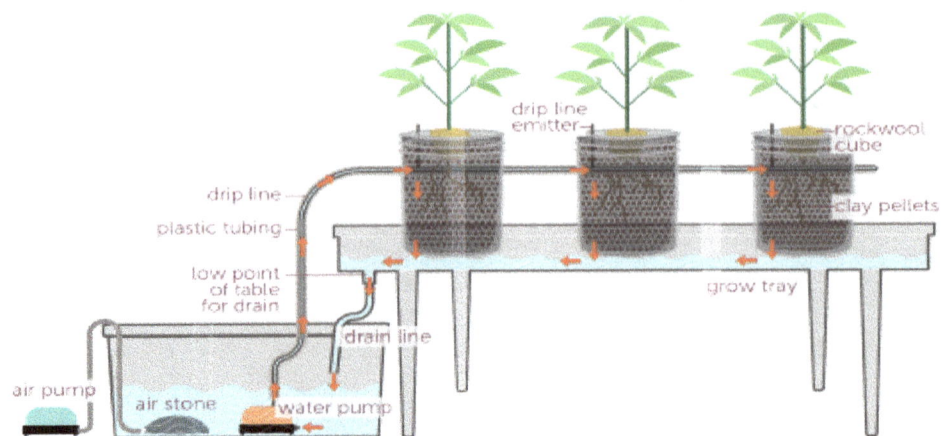

TYPES OF MARIJUANA

Marijuana is one of the only annual plants to have two different sexes. This means that plants can come in both male and female varieties, and even occasionally hermaphroditic varieties that have both male and female reproductive organs.

There are also three major species of marijuana:

- Indica: Relatively short and wide, with greener colors and round leaves that have marble-like patterns. Provides a heavy, body high.

- Sativa: Can grow taller, but are thinner with more pointed leaves that don't have patterns on them. Provides an energetic, cerebral high.

- Ruderalis: Lesser-known than the other two. Small plants, used primarily for making clothes, rope, etc.

Each of these types of marijuana has its own properties when it comes to actually using it.

One of the largest indicators of potency for a particular plant is its THC (tetrahydrocannabinol) content. This is essentially the stuff that provides the soothing, medicinal qualities that many people associate with cannabis. In general, most growers use indica, sativa, or hybrid varieties of the two. Ruderalis generally gets left out of any cannabis cultivation because it lacks a high amount of THC. Also, it should be pointed out that the female sex on the cannabis plant is most prized by growers because of its high THC content.

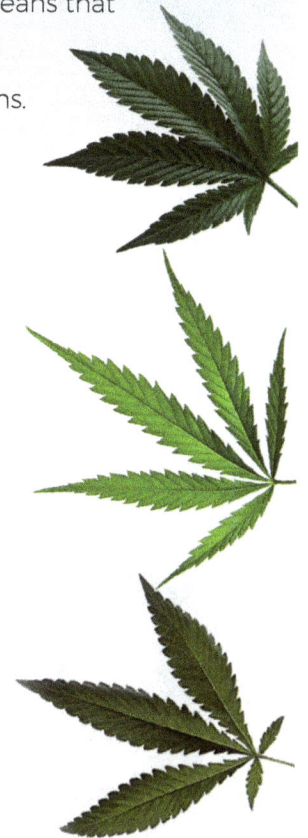

In general, the THC in female plants rises when the plant remains unpollinated. It will produce more flowers, more buds, and more THC resin, making the eventual smoke much more potent by the time of harvest. There are also plenty of other natural chemicals on a marijuana plant that influence the kind of high you receive.

These chemicals are referred to as cannabinoids, and they interact with your cognitive and physical functions to produce altered states of mind and being. Growing the plants under ideal conditions will promote high-quality THC production in your female plants. Indica/Sativa hybrids like Gorilla Glue, White Widow, Super Skunk and Girl Scout Cookies Extreme are very popular.

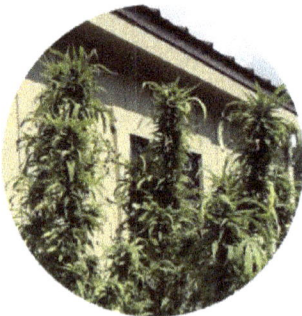
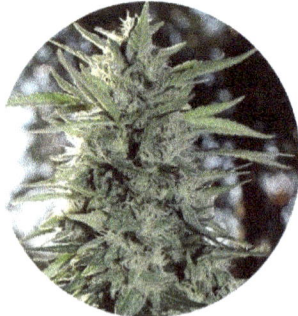
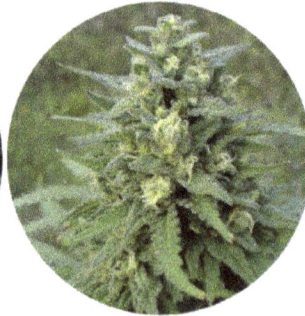
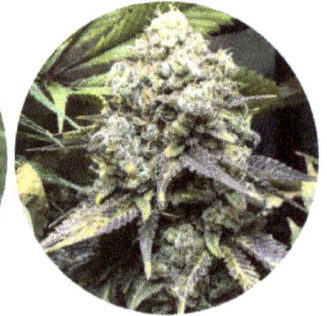

Gorilla Glue   White Widow   Super Skunk   Girl Scout Cookies Extreme

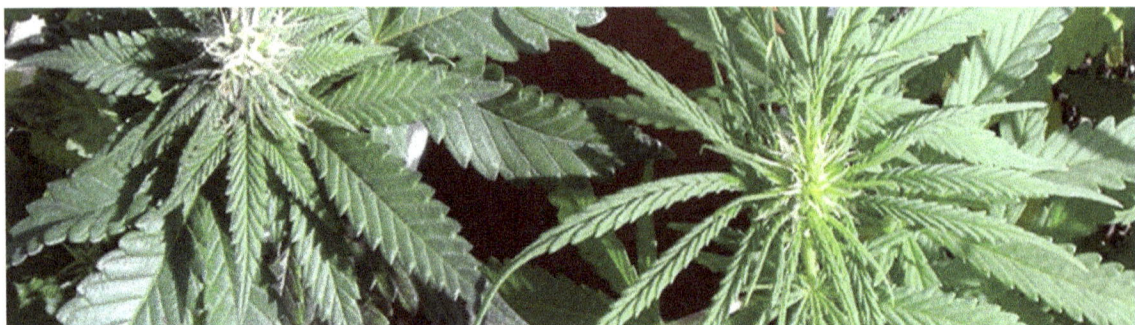

Indica, small and bushy   Sativa, tall and thin

MARIJUANA SEEDS

There are a number of ways to find marijuana seeds but, if you're in the United States, almost all of them are illegal. Of course, the most effective (and least expensive) way to get seeds is by receiving them from a friend. This will keep you off the radar of any law enforcement, and the seeds will be coming from a trusted source. There will be no surprises when it comes to the growth period or harvest time. Getting seeds from a fellow grower is an ideal scenario, but of course sometimes that isn't an option.

Another option you have at your disposal is buying seeds from a dealer. Of course, you'll need to have an in into the black market, and this option is really a toss-up when it comes to quality. It's possible to finish with some weird but very nice plants, but some of the seeds might be inert and won't grow to their full potential, if at all.

Your third option is to go through a seed bank. You can find a lot of these online, most of which are based out of the Netherlands or Canada where it's legal to sell marijuana seeds. Unfortunately, many Dutch seed banks refuse to ship to the US, and there is a decent possibility of getting ripped off in the end. There's minimal risk of being caught by any authorities because the seeds are packaged discreetly. Of course, if a postal employee mishandles the package, the seeds might come to you cracked or otherwise unusable. If you live near the border of Canada, you could also cross the border and find a physical seed bank that might be willing to sell to you.

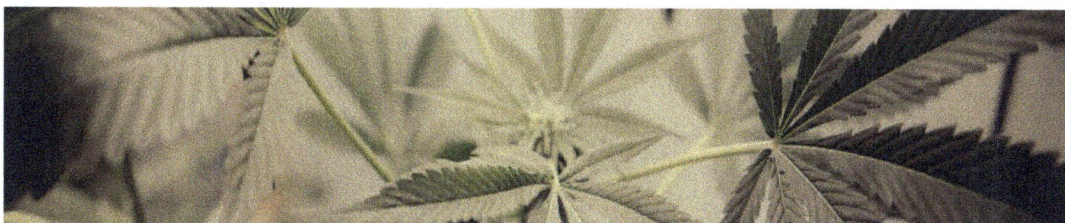

HEALTHY MARIJUANA SEEDS

For novice growers who have some experience with different marijuana strains, locating a favorite type is likely a priority. Most vendors categorize their seeds by strain. They might have unique names for their individual strains, but the species (i.e., indica, sativa, etc.) will reveal what you can expect from the smoke. In any event, it's important to find the seeds that best correlate to the smoking experience you desire.

Marijuana seeds can be a bit pricy, so make sure you purchase the right seeds!

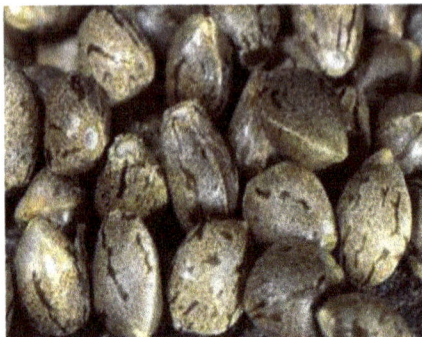

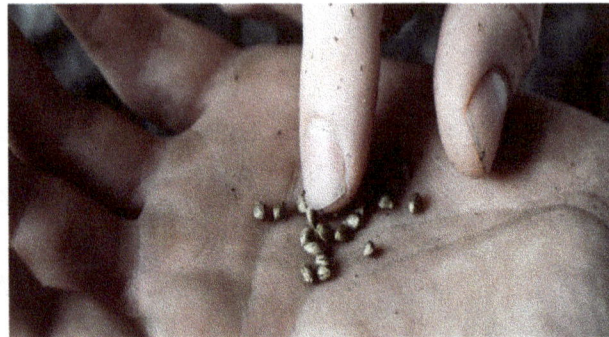

GROWING MARIJUANA

Obviously, obtaining seeds is only the first in a long line of steps that you must complete in order to start growing your marijuana plants. Before you start doing anything, you need to know where the growing will ultimately take place. Of course, there are two primary options: indoors or outdoors.

Growing marijuana isn't like picking up packages of pumpkin seeds at the grocery store and then throwing them into the ground. Many marijuana growers need to take stock of the feasibility of growing marijuana in the space they have to work with. For example, do you have enough space in your house to grow marijuana indoors? How many plants do you want to grow? Are you prepared for all of the unpredictabilities of being a grower? If you're growing marijuana outdoors, do you have a concealed location? How's the weather where you live? How's the soil?

The following sections of this e-book will explore the questions about indoor and outdoor growing.

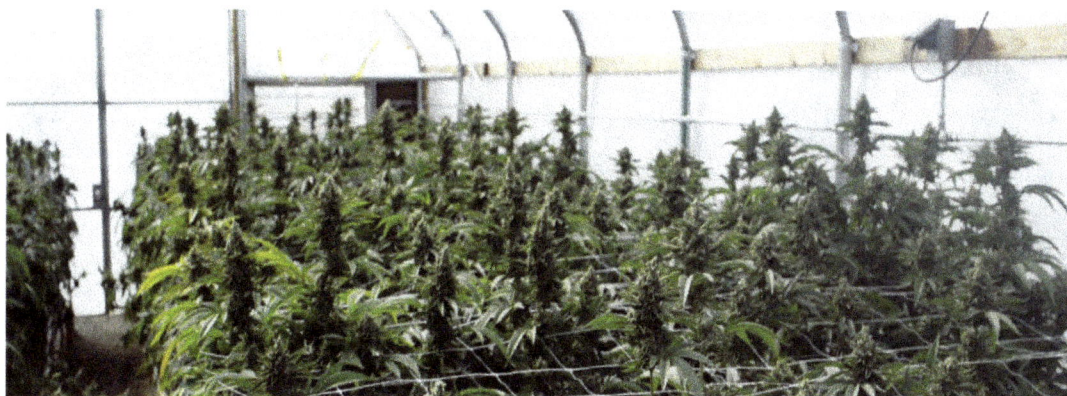

Indoor growing

For many people, growing marijuana indoors is the only option. Luckily, cannabis is a relatively versatile plant, and many varieties can be grown both indoors and out. Even so, you should check with the breeder (if at all possible) to see where the plants are best grown. Sometimes breeders develop seeds specifically for outdoor use. The last thing you want to do is grow marijuana plants indoors that were really meant for the great outdoors. If you grow your plants under the right circumstances, you can yield a lot of marijuana -- over a pound per square meter. Of course, temperature, air circulation, humidity, and plant care have to be perfect, but this can be controlled very well when growing indoors. No weather extremes or the neighbor's cat will damage your marijuana.

See here our top 3 Indoor strains!

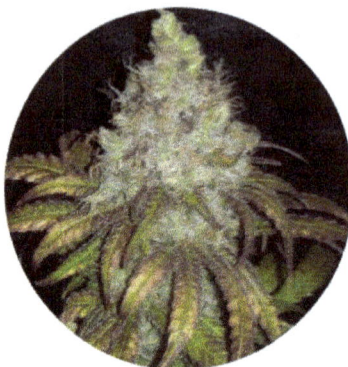

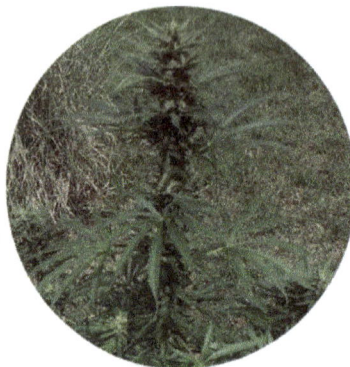

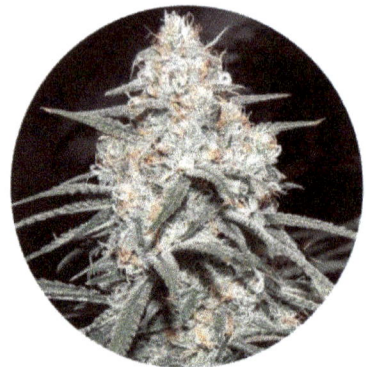

Grand Daddy Purple   LSD   Gelato

Lights

Lights often represent the lifeblood of plants that are grown indoors. Because any sunlight that they might receive is sparse, artificial light is valuable and necessary. Plants need the light to perform photosynthesis, which is vital for sugar and tissue production.

Many people who grow for personal use will use a closet space for their garden. Some can get away with using a guest bedroom that can't be seen from the outside and is rarely used otherwise. Regardless, every grower must assess the viability, both in terms of space and electrical capacity, of bringing in large amounts of lights.

Most growers limit their choices to one of the following three options: fluorescents, incandescents, and HID (high-intensity discharge) lamps. To save yourself some time and money, it's in your best interest to opt for HID lamps during the vegetative and flowering stage. These are sold as Metal Halide (MH) or High-Pressure Sodium (HPS) lamps and they are, without question, the best for your marijuana garden. Although they have a higher up-front cost than fluorescent or incandescent lights, their overall value is much greater in the long run because they don't require as much electricity as the other options, plus they are brighter also last much longer. Even if you're on a budget and don't want to throw away too much money up front, you must still factor in the cost of the electricity bill and bulb replacements.

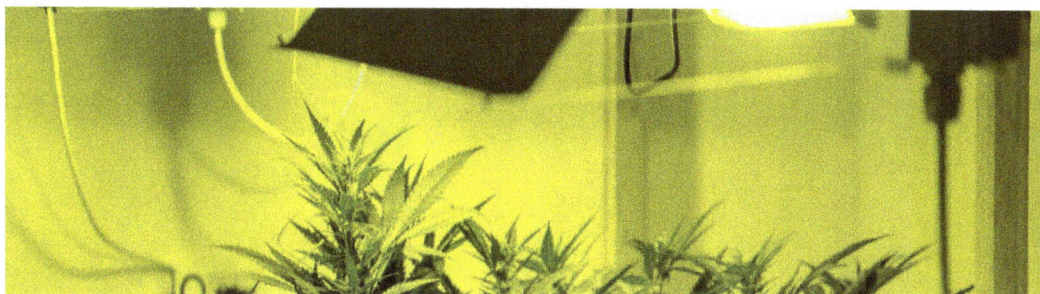

So, when it comes down to it, MH and HPS lamps represent a much better value and product overall. The plants will also need an even distribution of light so that growth is congruent. A lot of professional growers hook up a track system that allows the light(s) to be moved. With this technique, the plants receive an optimal amount of light without needing extra lights here and there.

For seedlings, an HPS light bulb can be too much, so many growers use fluorescent lights during germination. They don't produce a lot of heat and can be lowered to just four inches above the top leaves.

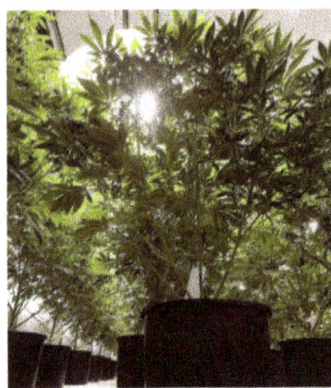

Reflective materials also helps enhance the amount of light that the plants receive. This can be as simple as lining the walls with aluminum foil or just painting the walls of the room with bright white paint. While mirrors undoubtedly look nice as decorations, they don't actually reflect as much light as other materials.

Large indoor gardens (and the light they require) place some heavy burdens on electricity, but personal growers really won't have any problems because they might only use a few hundred volts per hour. This usage would add, at the most, about $10 to the electric bill. Extensive growers, on the other hand, might be limited by the size of their circuit. For instance, older homes might only have a 15-amp circuit that can't maintain all the excess light that a large garden needs.

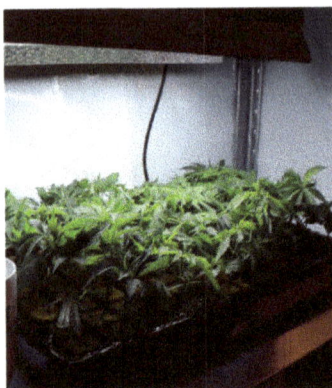

| Fluorescent light | Marijuana need a lot of light | HPS light |

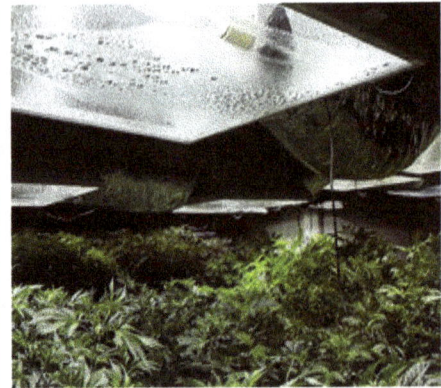

Germination

Once the lights are up, you can begin the process of germination. Germination essentially entails planting the marijuana seed and coercing it to sprout. If you don't provide it with the right environment, the seed will just remain a seed for the foreseeable future.

There are several methods that you can use to germinate your marijuana seeds, and every grower recommends something different. For the most part, the options are limited to either using soil (or another growing medium) or a wet paper towel.

Soil

Just by looking at these options, soil seems like it would be the most natural way of germinating a seed and, indeed, that is the case. Simply place the seed about 3 mm deep into the soil and keep the soil moist for about 7 days. This usually has around a 75% to 80% success rate in terms of getting seeds to germinate. This also depends on the seed quality.

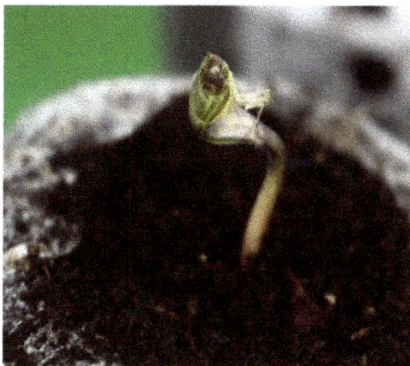

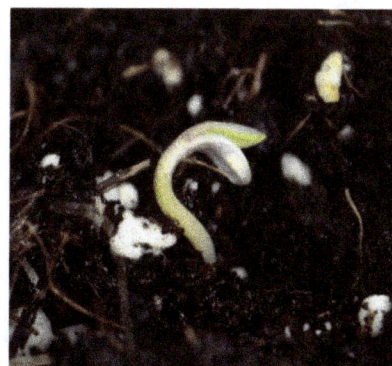

Wet paper method

The wet paper towel method is another method that is relatively simple. For this, you place the seed on a damp paper towel and fold the towel over it. In theory, the success rate with this method is around 80% to 90%, but it is more common for breakages to occur while transplanting. The seedling clearly won't be able to thrive in a paper towel, so transplanting is necessary, and it must be performed with great care.

Other options for germination include "propagation kits," which is just a fancy and more economical way to say "growing media for seeds." These include Rockwool cubes and have a similar success rate when compared to the paper towel trick. You can find these kits at many garden centers.

Still, the easiest method for any beginner is just to use soil. Transplanting will not be necessary, and it really is the most natural way to get your seeds to germinate adequately. When transplanting the seedlings at such an early age, you run the risk of "shocking" the plants. This will either stunt their growth or kill them altogether, so it makes sense to just stick with using soil until you get comfortable enough as a grower to use something else.

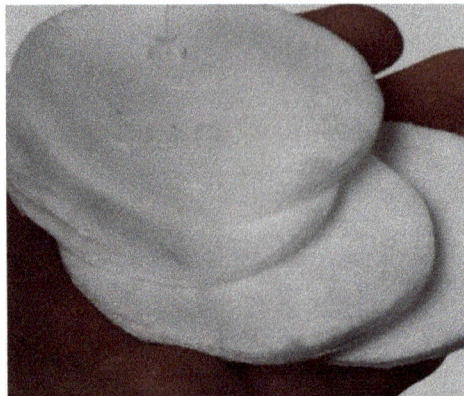

Soaking in water

I advise to use this method because it has the highest success rate in our experience.

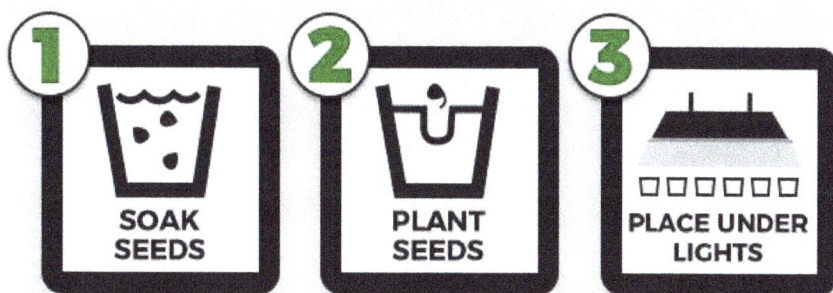

1 SOAK SEEDS

Soak your seeds in water. They will sproute a tail between 24 to 72 hours.

2 PLANT SEEDS

Put your seeds in a 1/2 inch hole in soil in little pots, gently cover with soil.

3 PLACE UNDER LIGHTS

Place pots under a 36 watts CFL tube at 2 inch distance from plants.

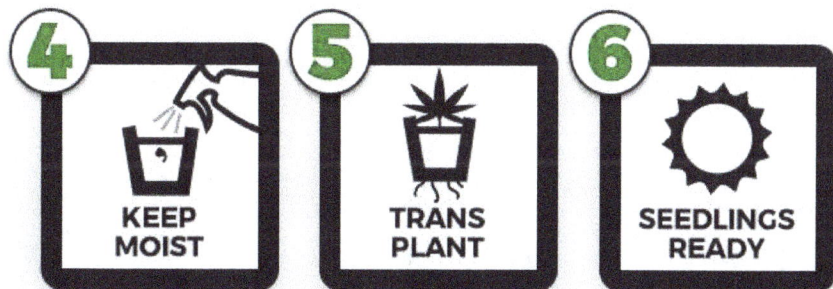

4 KEEP MOIST

Keep the soil moist and spray water with a plant sprayer twice a day

5 TRANS PLANT

After 2 to 3 weeks roots may grow out of the bottom, time to transplant to bigger pots

6 SEEDLINGS READY

Once the plants are 8 to 12 inch high they're ready to move outdoor or under HPS/LED lights.

I've met many growers over the years, and everybody has their own way of germinating seeds. Some prefer soil, others rockwool or peat pots. What is your favorite way of germinating seeds?

Germination soil

This brings up an obvious question: "What kind of soil should I use for germination?" At many garden centers, you will find soils that are marketed specifically as "germination soils". Nothing really separates these soils from more conventional soils except that they have certain nutrients and don't contain any composted material. Look for soils that have an NPK (Nitrogen-Phosphorus-Potassium) ratio of around 5:1:1 or 8:4:4. Really, any soil with more nitrogen than the other two nutrients will be adequate for germinating marijuana seeds.

The containers you place the soil in are also relatively important. It's common for growers to use buckets that can hold between 2 and 5 gallons because the root system in a marijuana plant can become quite extensive. Smaller containers will work for the germination and seedling period, but the plants will need to be transplanted later. Thus, it makes sense to plant the marijuana seeds and leave the plants in a single 2- to 5-gallon bucket for the majority of their lives. This gives the roots adequate room to grow and thrive while also providing a perfect environment for nutrients and a satisfactory reservoir of water. Also, leaving them in buckets makes them easily transportable.

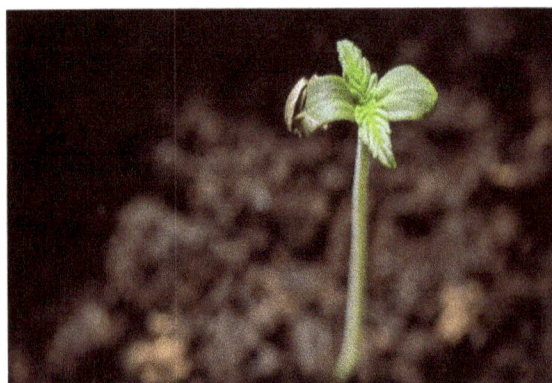

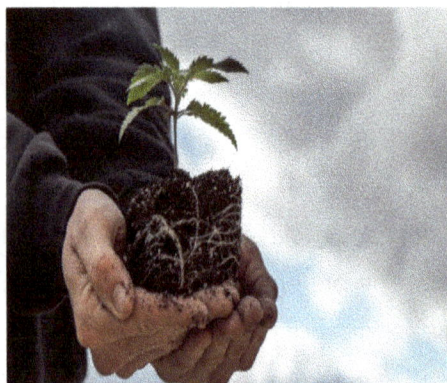

Depending on the intensity of the lights you use, the plants will need about 25 to 35 watts per square foot. The seeds won't need light to germinate right away, but it's common for growers to turn the lights on after sowing the seeds to warm the soil and promote germination. It's also a good idea to keep the lights on and ready for when the first sprouts appear out of the soil.

A few other things to take into account are the pH balance and the actual texture of the soil. You can feasibly use the same soil throughout the life of the plant if you ensure that water can drain properly (soil texture) and the soil maintains a good pH balance (between 6.0 and 8.0). The texture is particularly important because soils should neither be too dry nor too moist. Moist soils that have an almost muddy consistency reduce the amount of oxygen that can reach the roots. As long as the roots can "breathe" and still maintain adequate water uptake, the soil should be fine.

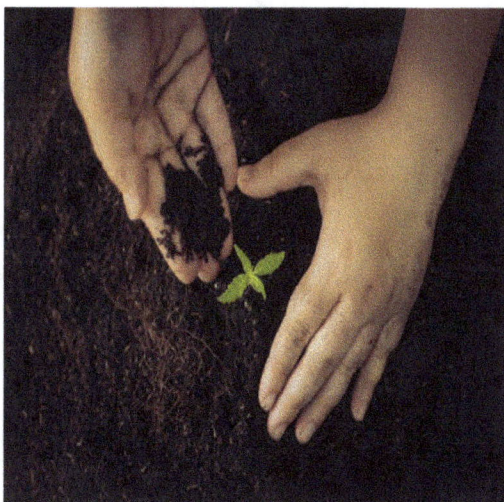

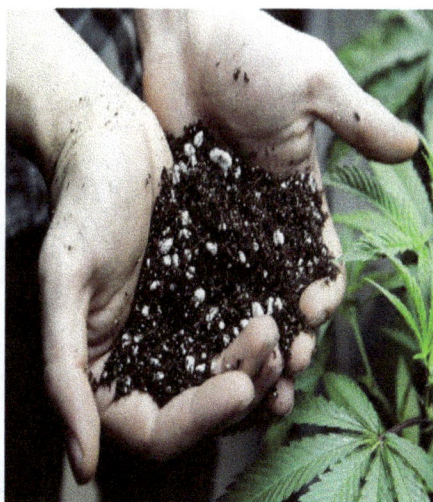

Light Cycle and Distance from Plants

Perhaps the best thing about growing marijuana indoors is that you have more control over virtually every aspect of the growing process.

While the seeds themselves won't need light initially, they will certainly need some light when they produce visible sprouts. Light acts as their sustenance during this period of time, and it can affect the plants later in life if they are deprived of the valuable light they require. This assumes, of course, that the soil, nutrient quality, and watering regimen are all adequate as well.

At this delicate stage, the lights should be somewhat close to the marijuana plants. In fact, dropping them down to about four inches away from the soil is ideal if you use fluorescent lights. The light cycle should also be relatively consistent at around 16 to 18 hours of light per day. This will be the light cycle for a majority of the plant's life, but it can be hard to maintain a reliable schedule. To remedy this, you can purchase an automatic timer, which only costs about $8 and will let you focus on other things.

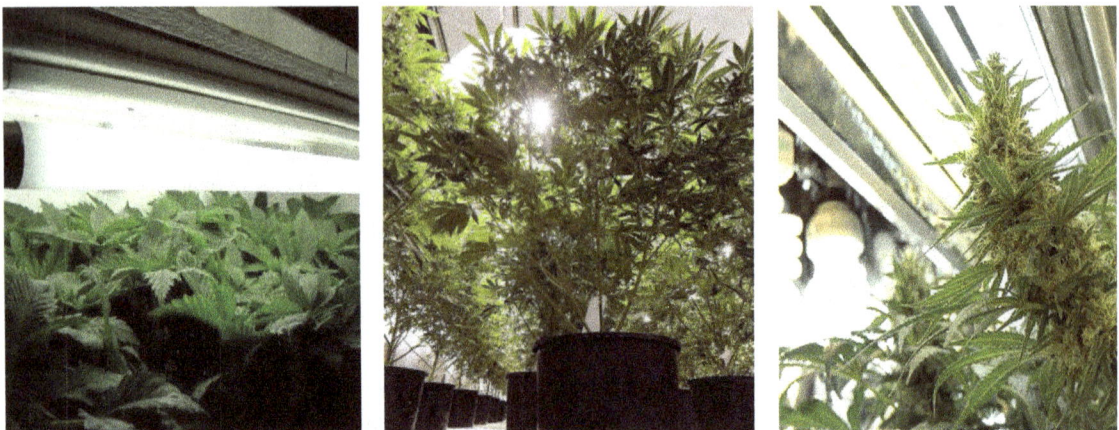

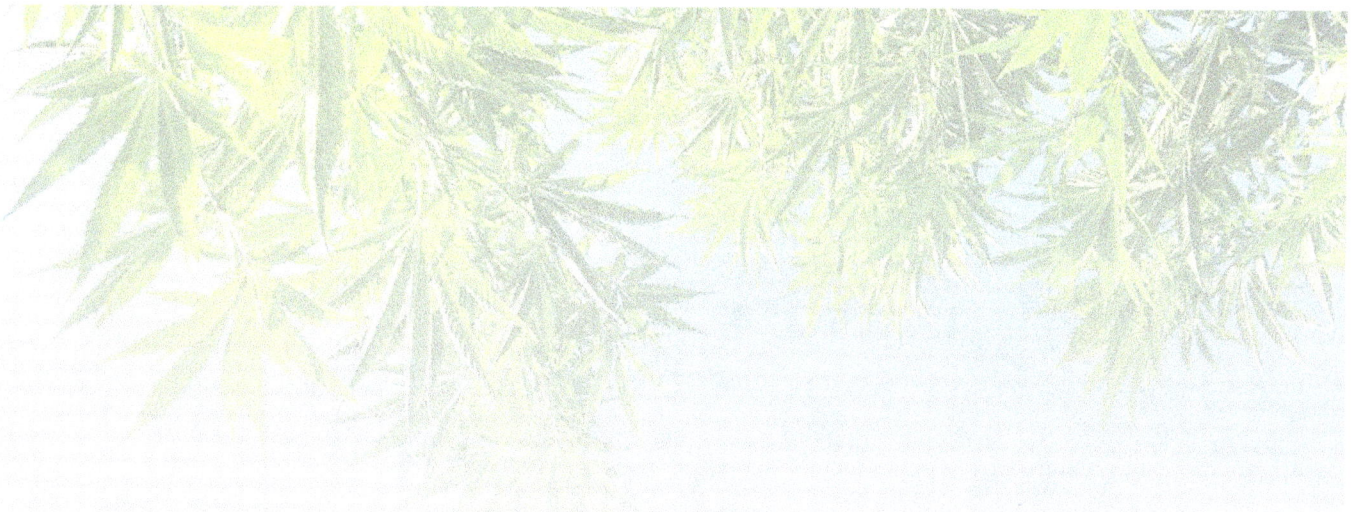

Depending on the particular strain, some plants could stand to use a more intensive light regimen. Cannabis really tends to absorb light voraciously because it is a high-energy plant. Some marijuana growers have been known to expose their plants to a light cycle with a full 24 hours of light. Most growers won't have to go to those extremes, but you may need to increase the light cycle to over 18 hours at some point if you want to improve growth. Of course, an automatic light timer can make this considerably easier, and some lights actually come installed with a timer.

As the marijuana plant ages and starts to grow, the lights should still remain as close to the leaves as possible without damaging them. The instructions on the lights might tell you to keep them at a certain distance from the plants, but cannabis requires a lot of light energy to thrive. In fact, with lower output bulbs, you can place the lights 2 to 4 inches away from the tops of the leaves. For higher output bulbs, you can place them 4 to 6 inches from the tops of the leaves.

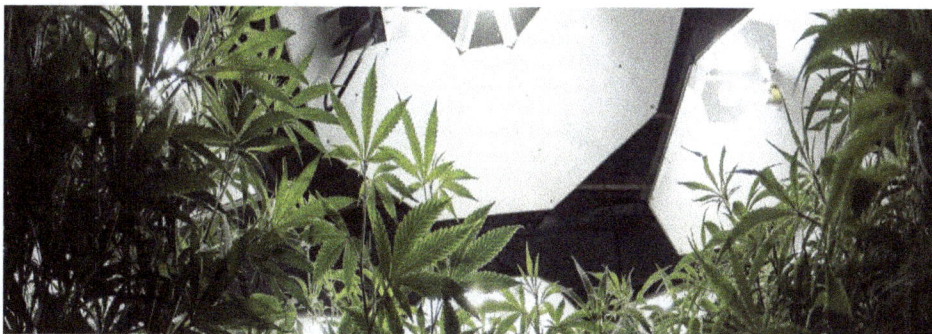

Watering

Every living thing on the planet requires water in some form, but, when working with marijuana, extra caution should be exercised. During the germination period, avoid overwhelming the marijuana plant with moisture. The top layer of soil should be kept moist, but even then it's best to only use a few spritzes of water from a spray bottle. When the plant actually sprouts, keep the area near the stem dry. This is because moist conditions around the stem are often conducive to stem rot.

At this stage (and, really, any stage) it's relatively easy to overwater marijuana plants. Using excessive water can cause significant issues with the soil and place stress on the plants. As mentioned previously, the soil should not be too wet. If you make the soil soggy by over-watering it, the roots will essentially drown due to a lack of oxygen.

This is particularly true when watering small marijuana seedlings in large pots. These plants won't need to be watered as much as bigger plants because they won't need to take in as much water.

Unfortunately, it can be hard to tell if you are overwatering your plants because the symptoms of overwatering and underwatering are exactly the same (i.e. the leaves will droop). One way to check is by inspecting the moisture level of the soil. You can do this by merely touching the soil with your hand. If the soil feels damp, then holding off on watering your plants is the best course of action. It will still have plenty of water to draw from in the soil if it is clearly moist. If the soil is dry, then adding more water is advisable. As the plants grow, they will require more and more water to quench their thirst.

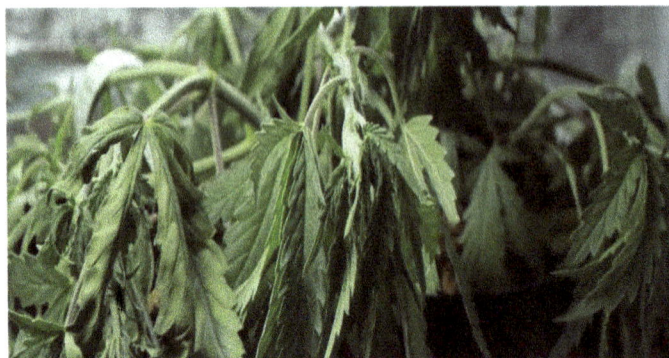

Overwatered

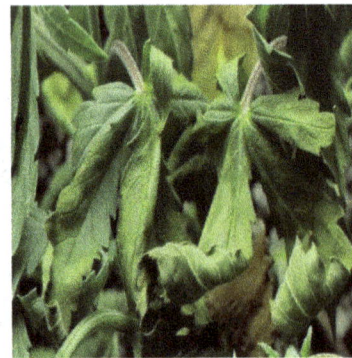

Underwatered

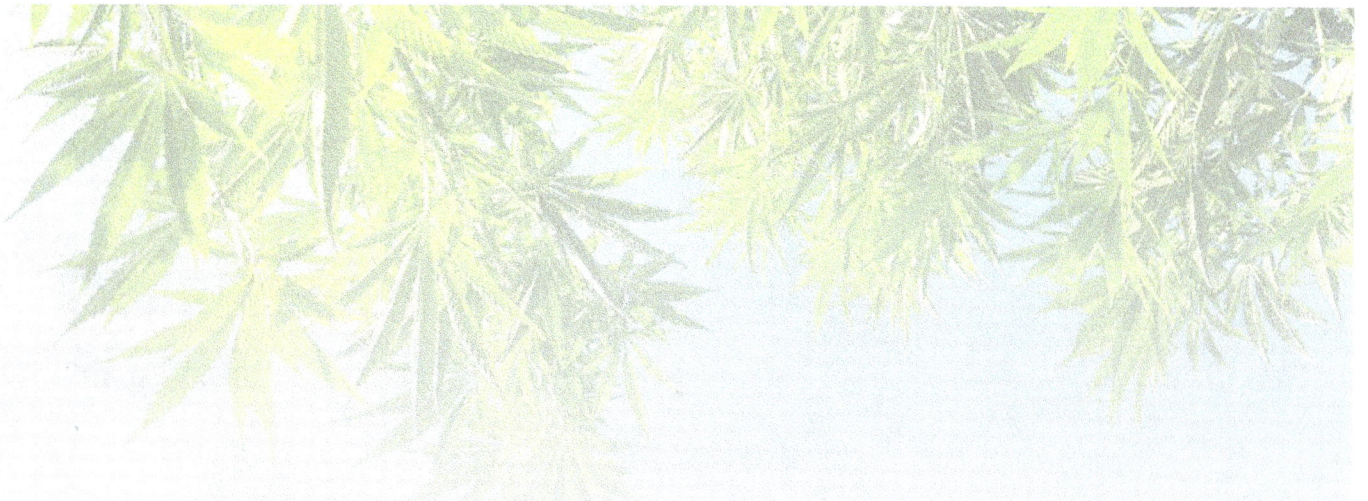

Overall, keeping the soil exceptionally moist or exceptionally dry for any long period of time will not be good for the plants. In fact, it actually needs to alternate between moist and dry to provide better aeration in the soil.

Tap water is frequently used to grow marijuana, but many growers have concerns about its viability. Some municipal water systems put a lot of chlorine in the water which could kill beneficial bacteria around the plant. In general, chlorine isn't going to be a huge problem, and many plants grow and thrive using chlorinated water. Some solutions that are normally used for fish tanks can also work for growing a marijuana garden. Try adding sodium to the tap water prior to watering. The sodium then bonds with chlorine in the water to make sodium chloride (a.k.a. salt). This won't harm the plant but, if used in excess, the soil could become too saline.

It's also possible for your water supply to be infected with other minerals, which is a condition known as hard water. While hard water might be detrimental to your plumbing over an extended period of time, it won't have any negative effects on the plants. In fact, the minerals in the water actually help promote growth by adding extra nutrients. It is advisable to stay away from artificial water softeners during the growing period because they tend to put excessive amounts of sodium in the water supply, making it unsafe for the soil and the plant. They also use a lot of other artificial additives that might not be good for your plant later on.

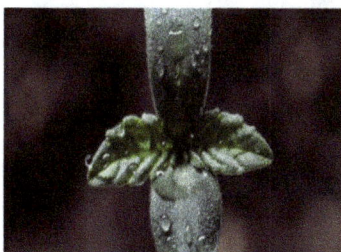

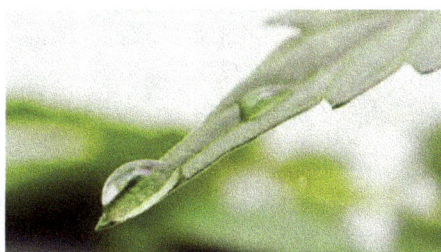

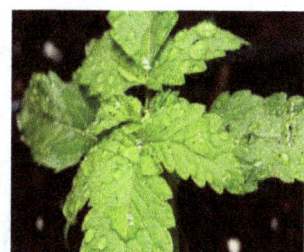

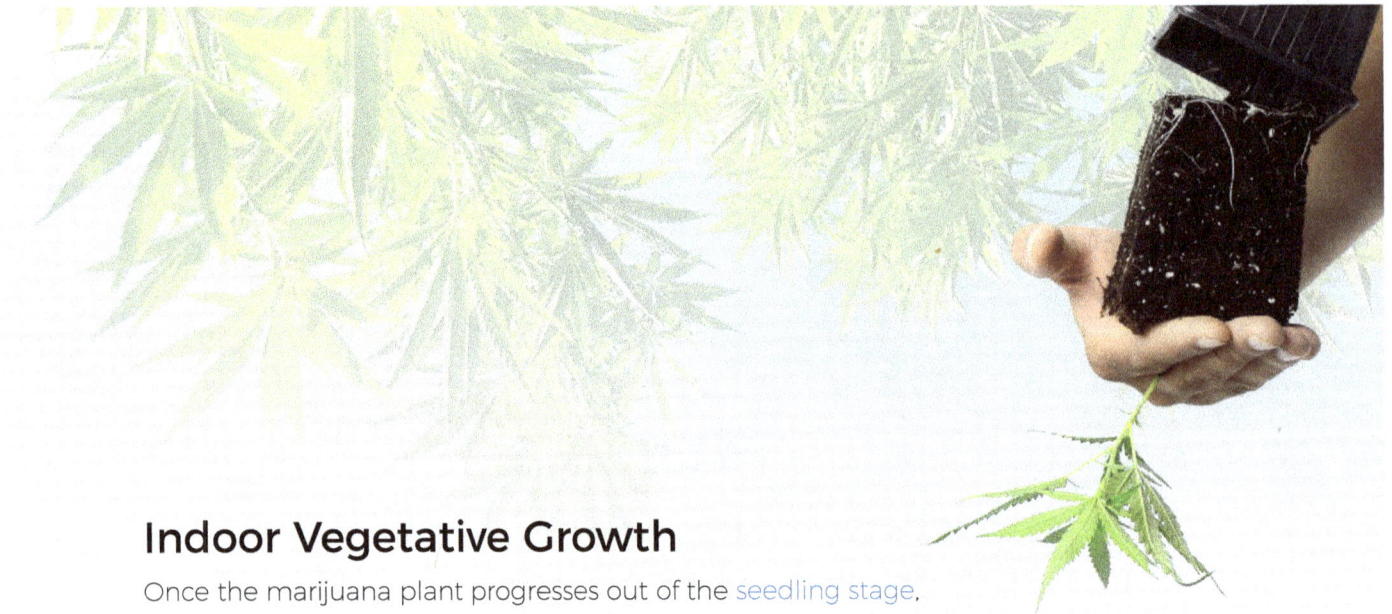

Indoor Vegetative Growth

Once the marijuana plant progresses out of the seedling stage, it will enter the vegetative growth period. During this time, the growth rate will increase by leaps and bounds, with more leaves and branches appearing. The seedlings will also finally start looking like actual marijuana plants.

Transplanting

Marijuana plants that were germinated in small pots will need to be transplanted to larger ones as soon as the vegetative growth starts kicking in. If the containers are too small for the plants, they can quickly become rootbound and begin to lose vigor (or even die). The key is, of course, to transplant them before that happens.

Of course, the transplanting process should be treated with a lot of care because transplant shock is common. You can avoid transplant shock if you treat the process with extreme caution. Before you do anything, make sure the soil is moist so that nothing will be jarred out of place. Then, insert a spade (or even a large spoon) into the soil about 1 inch away from the plant's stem. Make sure that you don't damage the roots and that you take out a large enough clump to do the transplant. You should have a previously prepared hole in the new soil. It should be dug in such a way that the seedling will be at the same height.

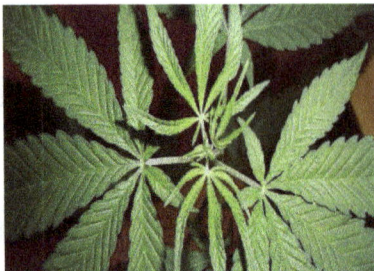

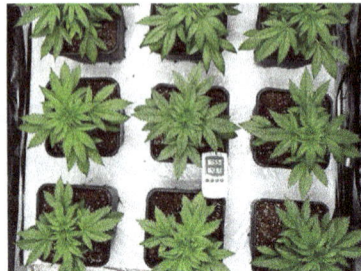

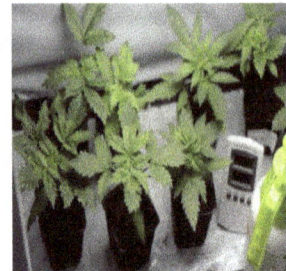

Place the plant into the hole and cover it as best as you can with the new soil. Then, moisten the soil so that the transplant and the host soil meld nicely together. If you do this carefully and correctly, you won't have to worry about the plants suffering from any transplant shock, and they will continue to grow like normal. I transplant my plants when the first root tips grow out the bottom of the pot.

Vegetative Growth Techniques

From this point on, the plants will primarily live out their lives in vegetative growth. It is important to make sure that you provide them with all the proper environmental conditions during this stage to promote growth, higher yields, and potency. One of the benefits of growing marijuana indoors is that you can manipulate the conditions exactly as you see fit without having to worry about environmental factors.

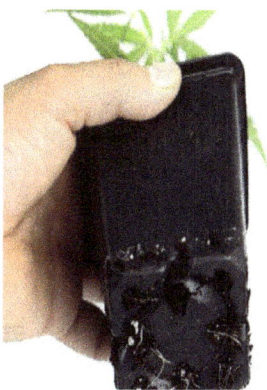

Squeeze pot and hold upside down

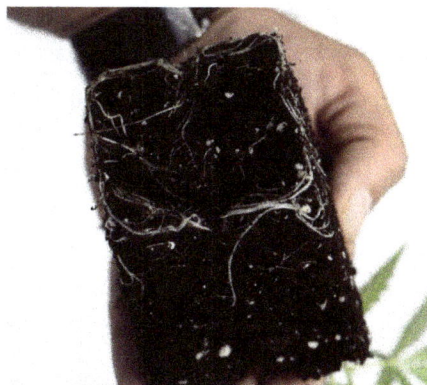

Beware of becoming rootbound

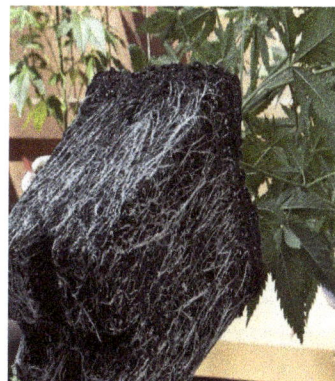

Rootbound

Water and Lighting

We've already seen how plants should be watered and how much light they should receive. During the vegetative growth period, the plants are likely going to become "thirstier" and require more water as they get larger. The same rules still apply when it comes to watering: don't severely overwater and don't severely underwater. Many growers develop patterns for watering their marijuana plants. For instance, you might water one day, skip watering for two days, and then water again.

It really depends on the plants themselves. You need to pay close attention to exactly how dry the soil gets after a few days. If the soil is still moist, then you can probably continue with the same pattern, but, if it dries out significantly before the next scheduled watering, you should increase the rate at which you're watering the marijuana plants.

When it comes to light, marijuana requires a lot of it. In fact, it is feasible to keep the lights on 24 hours per day to achieve the maximum growth potential. Adjustable light tracks are ideal when you have a large grow room and little electricity so that you can move the lights around to every part of your garden. This way, every plant gets intense amounts of high-quality light.

Try to keep a sharp eye on the distance between the lights and the top of the plant canopy; 20 to 30 inches is usually perfect. The accelerated rate at which the plants tend to grow will cause them to inch closer to the lights almost on a daily basis. So, be sure to place the lights close enough so that they provide adequate light energy, but far enough away that they don't burn the tips of the leaves.

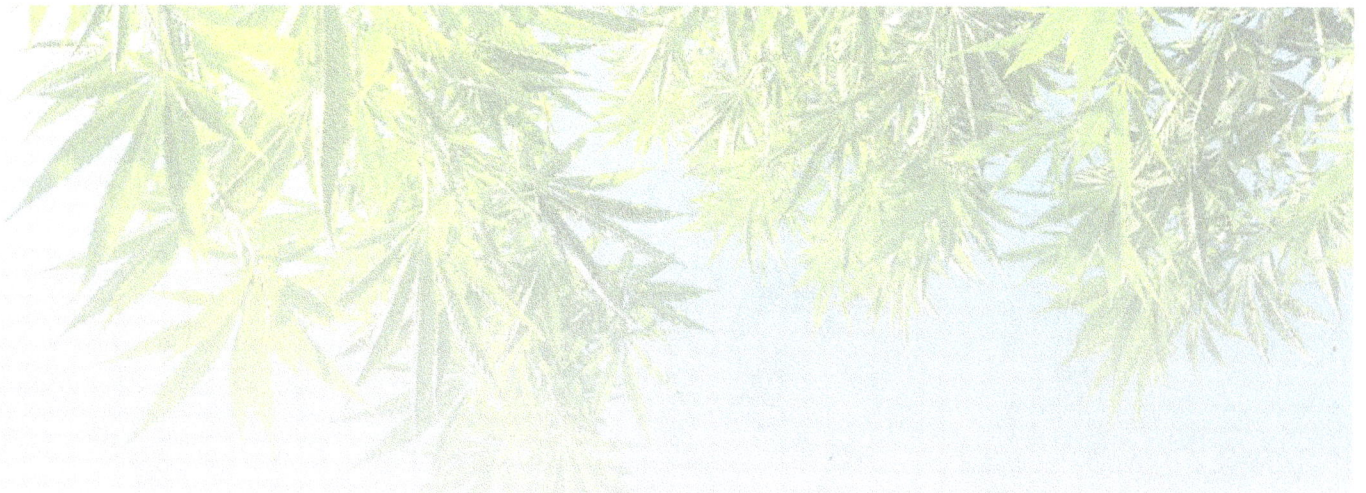

If you want to avoid this, install an air-cooled or water-cooled system that will essentially reduce the heat that the lights produce. Electric light bulbs produce both light and heat whenever they are turned on. Of course, if you let them go unchecked, they can create incredibly hot temperatures. But, if you want to make use of all the light they have to offer, a cooling system will allow the lights to get closer and work better in the long run.

It should also be noted that certain lights emit different color spectrums. When we talk about visible light, we're referring to all the colors that we can see which is often represented by "ROYGBIV" (red, orange, yellow, green, blue, indigo, and violet). Marijuana tends to thrive under light that is strong in the red spectrum. This promotes photosynthesis, which is vital for tissue production during vegetative growth. High-pressure sodium (HPS) lamps produce the most light in the red spectrum (and the most light in general) and are often the best choice during virtually every stage of the growing process.

Using anything that is high in the green spectrum will produce wilted, unproductive plants in general. This is largely because the plants reflect green light entirely, which is why they are green in color themselves.

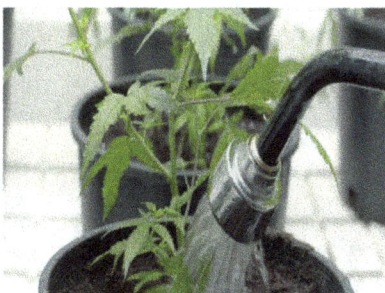

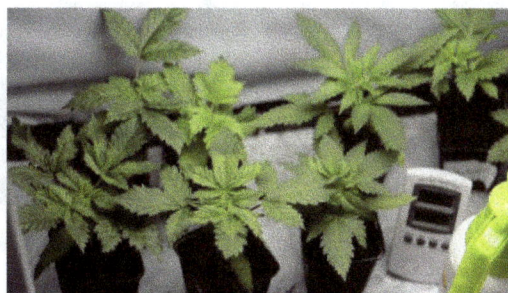

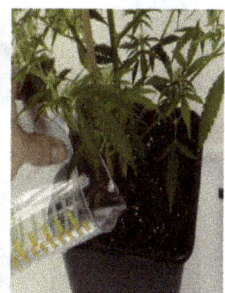

Vegetative stage

SOIL CONTROL

When you have an indoor marijuana garden you have more control over the soil, so you'll need to keep an eye on it. Marijuana prefers to grow in a nutrient-rich soil that has a neutral pH of around 7.0. Sometimes, however, the pH in the soil can shift quite far out of the acceptable ranges of 6.0 to 8.0. In such cases, you may need to take drastic measures to ensure that the soil does not end the life of your plants.

When pH levels fluctuate, it is often caused by chemical contamination. A soil flush can reduce contamination and balance the pH. However, this is generally not a recommended procedure, although it is sometimes necessary. A soil flush should only be used as a last resort when trying to keep your marijuana plant alive. To do it, place your entire plant, pot included, in a sink. From there, turn on the faucet and let the water run through the soil so that it eliminates any of the contaminants that might have been harming the plant. The danger of this method is a risk of killing the plant by oversaturation. Too much water is as bad as too many nutrients. But, sometimes flushing the soil is the only way to ensure that additives don't kill your marijuana plants.

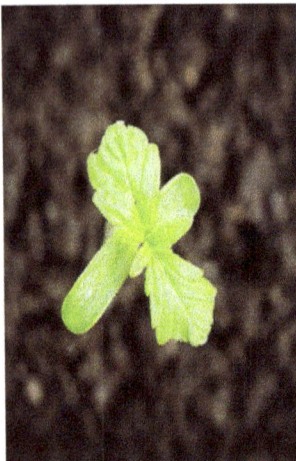

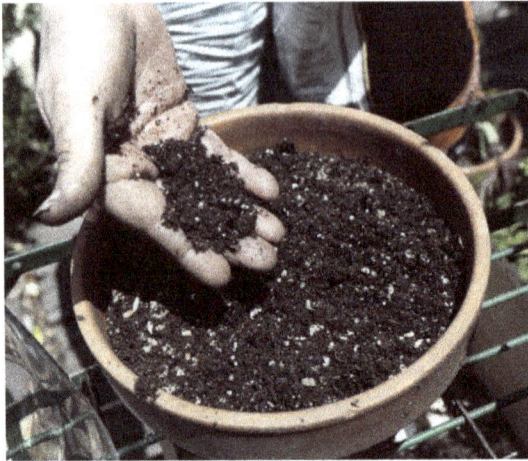

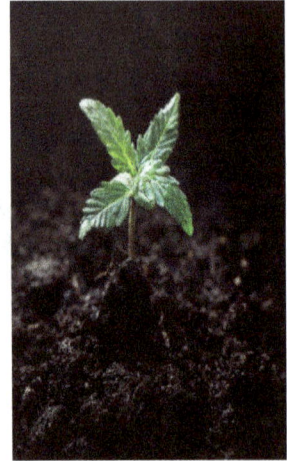

For less severe issues, there are other options. If your soil's pH level drops below the recommended 6.0 and becomes too acidic, then you can simply add some lime to the soil the next time you water it. This should raise the pH back into an acceptable range between 6 and 8. If the soil is above 8 and, therefore, too alkaline, you might consider adding a mixture of cottonseed meal, lemon peels, and ground coffee.

Some fertilizers are also made to be highly acidic and can lower your soil's alkalinity if applied. In any event, it's always a good idea to keep checking the pH balance of your soil; otherwise, you could be in for a disappointing surprise. Here you can see pH problems, on the left the pH level is too high, on the right the pH level is too low.

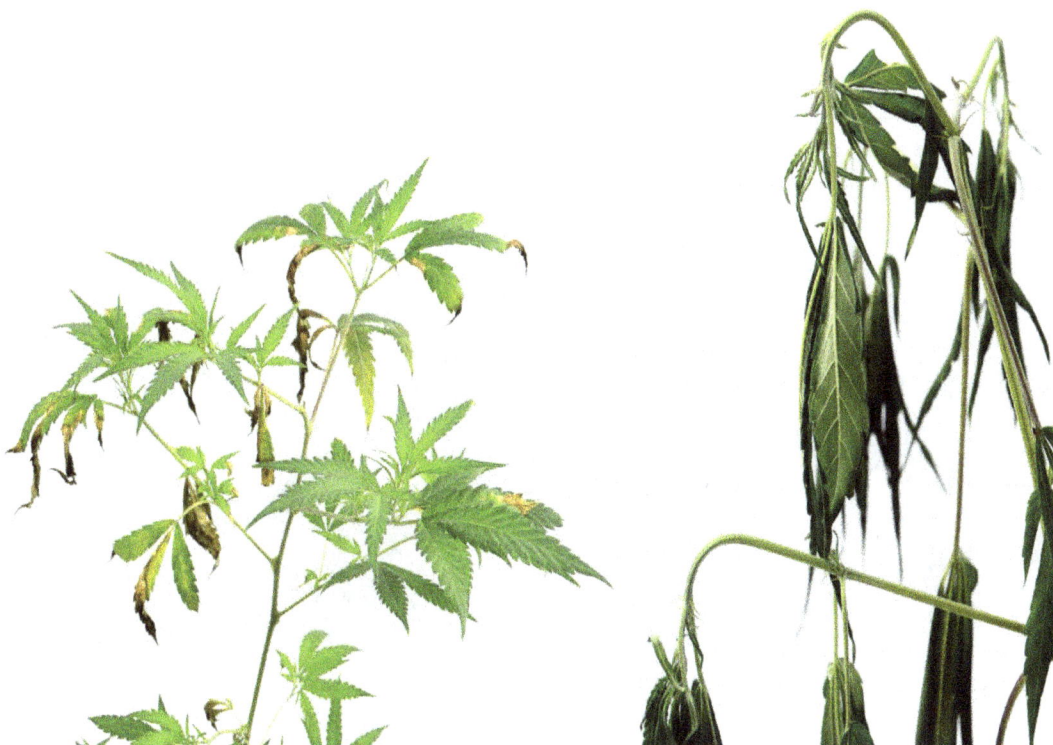

NUTRIENTS AND FEEDING

Of course, the primary cause of any significant irregularities in soil pH comes from the nutrients that you apply. Unlike standard dirt, soil for growing marijuana should be infused with nutrients. Sometimes, you can produce an adequate amount of nutrients just by combining certain fertilizers. But, in many cases, you will "water in" the nutrients using a solution. Of course, if you accidentally include too many nutrients, you could wind up making the soil toxic (and then you will have to flush it out to fix it). Your water should have the proper pH as well. Professional growers use water with a pH of around 6.

In any event, all plants need nutrients to thrive, and providing them with those nutrients can ensure that your work pays off in the end. We have already mentioned "NPK" (nitrogen, phosphorus, and potassium) as the three major nutrients for marijuana growers. Other essential chemicals for the cannabis plant include Calcium (Ca), Magnesium (Mg), and Sulfur (S).

During vegetative growth, the fertilizing solution should have a concentration of N that is higher than or equal to both P and K. Again, you can use fertilizer if you want, however, it should be mixed in with the soil before beginning the growth process.

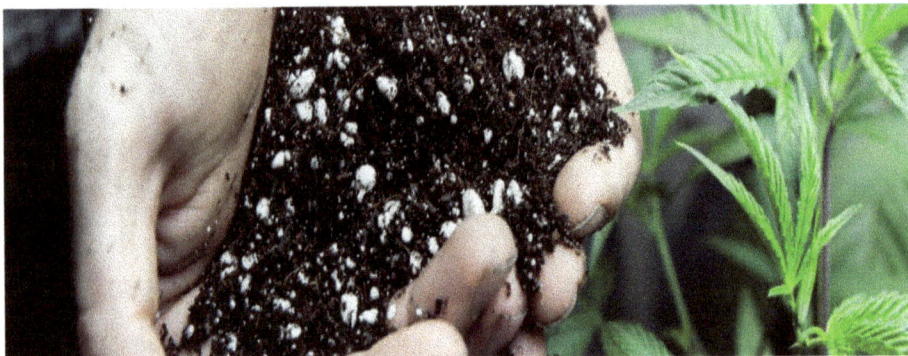

There are also solutions that can be used for "feeding" the plant instead of mixing it into the soil; but keep in mind the fact that the plant won't need to be fed that frequently. In fact, you only need to feed it about once every week if everything is going well. Note: you should never give your plants undiluted nutrients. Marijuana plants "burn" easily from full-strength nutrients. Instead, dilute the solution to around 50% so that you don't have to use a soil flush later.

In general, you might not be able to notice whether or not your plants are fully absorbing the nutrients. In fact, in most cases, the nutrient uptake will be the least of your worries. As long as the soil is good and you continue to use the same regimen, you should be all right. Many growers keep several diluted solutions on hand to make growing just a little bit easier. One of those should be an NPK solution where N has the most prominent concentration. This should be used for vegetative growth. Another should be an NPK solution in which the P has the highest concentration (used for the flowering stage). You can also keep a couple of bottles of diluted micronutrient solution if your plants need extra help along the way.

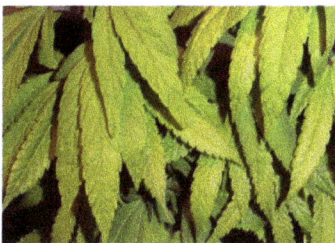

Nitrogen deficiency

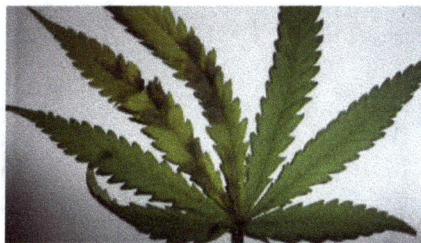

Phosphorus deficiency

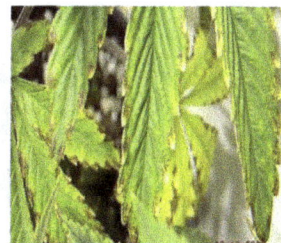

Potassium deficiency

Pruning

Pruning marijuana plants can be both a logistical necessity and something that helps produce more buds when it comes time to harvest. Many indoor growers will want to keep their plants 'in check' if they start to grow too high due to a lack of vertical space in their grow room. For the most part, indoor plants don't grow as large as outdoor plants, but they will need to be kept at bay if they start to grow really tall. Snipping off the top stem will also force the plant to create more branches and grow broader instead of taller. This way, although you may lose vertical height, you probably won't lose any of your yield.

If your goal is to ensure uniform growth, cutting the shoots and leaves won't really harm the plant if done in moderation. However, you don't want to get too carried away with this because cutting too many shoots and leaves can make it hard for the plant to regrow. You have to give it some time to recuperate before cutting off a significant amount of leaves or shoots.

For many growers, this might seem like a waste of perfectly adequate leaves and shoots, but during vegetative growth, the shoots are the most potent part of the plant. They can produce a high-quality smoke that will at least get you a little buzzed. The leaves can also be used in cooking preparations for potent edibles.

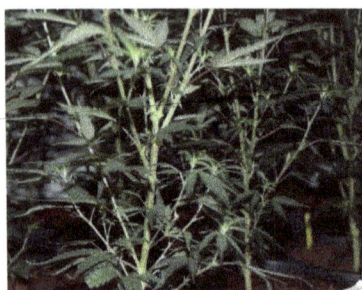

Before pruning

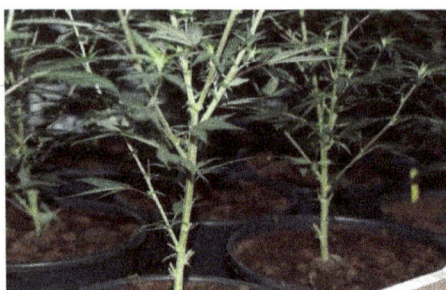

After pruning

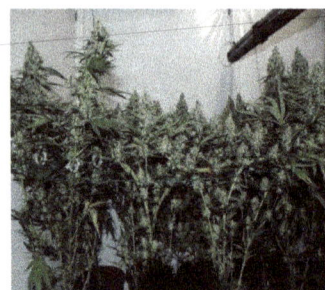

After few weeks

OTHER ENVIRONMENTAL FACTORS

While it might seem obsessive, the vegetative growth period requires complete attention to detail on every aspect of the plant's development. Neglecting even one issue could end up causing detrimental effects in terms of your plant's ability to thrive and produce excellent bud.

Air

As with most living things, fresh air is something precious. Opening up a window or installing a fan system in the room can help provide your plants with some much-needed fresh air. Of course, if it is particularly cold outside, it's probably not a good idea to keep the window open for too long, even if it's your only means of refreshing the air. The cold outside will stunt plant growth and make it difficult for you to help them recover.

Temperature

The temperature of the plants and the grow room is also something that needs to be monitored and regulated. The average temperature for a grow room should be around 75°F. Even so, cannabis is remarkably adaptive and will produce buds in lower or higher temperatures. If the temperature drops to extreme lows or rises to extreme highs, then you could be in for a surprise when it comes to the quality of your plants. Although cannabis can survive at temperatures as low as 50 to 55°F, it will not produce the most potent bud in those conditions. In general, keeping the room at about 75°F is your best bet. In reality, plants will grow slightly better at slightly higher temperatures, but it might be difficult to maintain those higher temperatures. You might also need to counteract the extra heat by watering the plants more to cool down the roots.

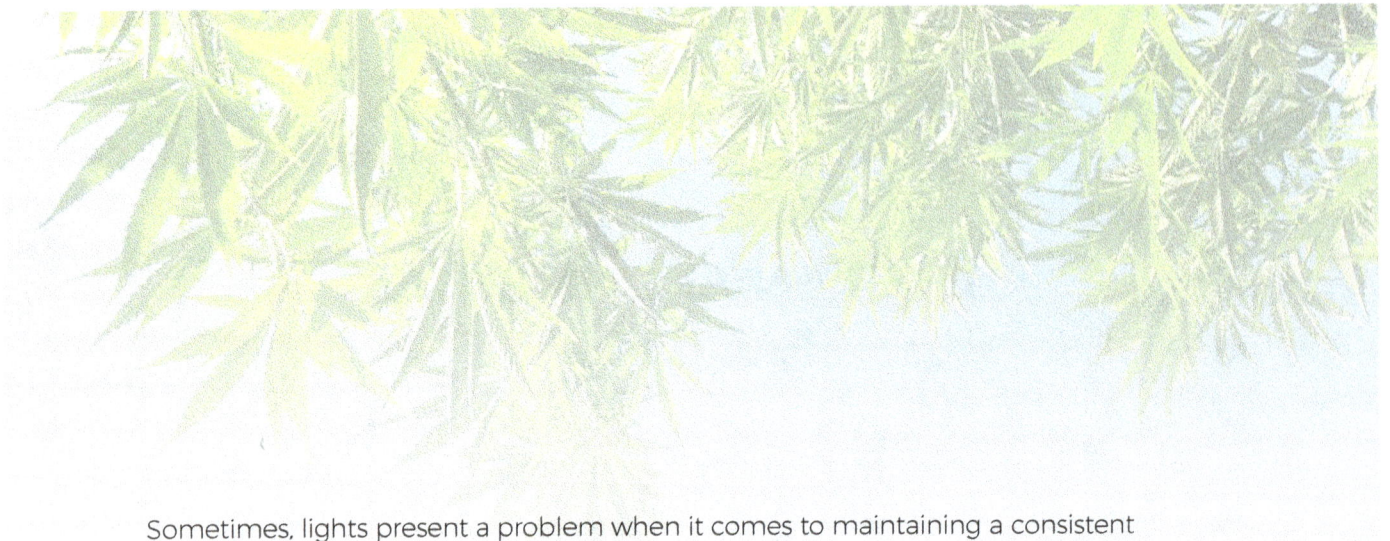

Sometimes, lights present a problem when it comes to maintaining a consistent temperature. Lights that produce a great deal of heat can give the room a sweltering feel and cause the plants to dry up or burn. If this is a problem, then you might want to install an air- or water-cooled system to alleviate the extra heat. You can even install an air conditioner if it is cost effective for your grow room. Most homes maintain an average temperature that is ideal for growing marijuana, but it's essential to monitor the temperature on a daily basis to ensure that your plants are being taken care of properly.

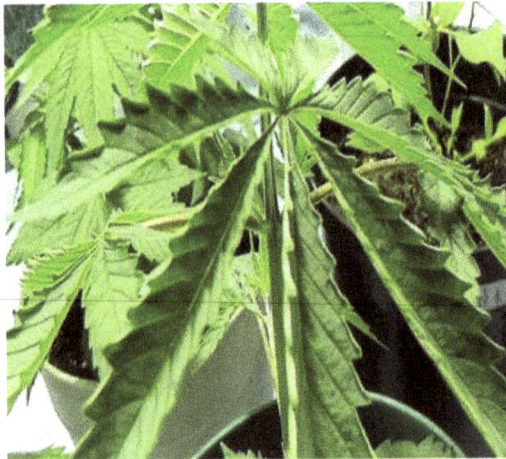

Too hot, curling leaves

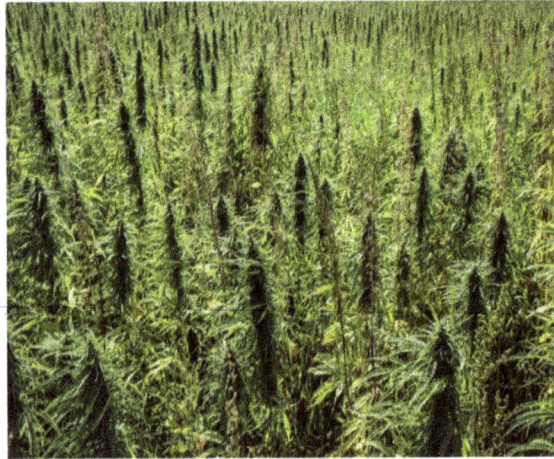

Perfect temperature

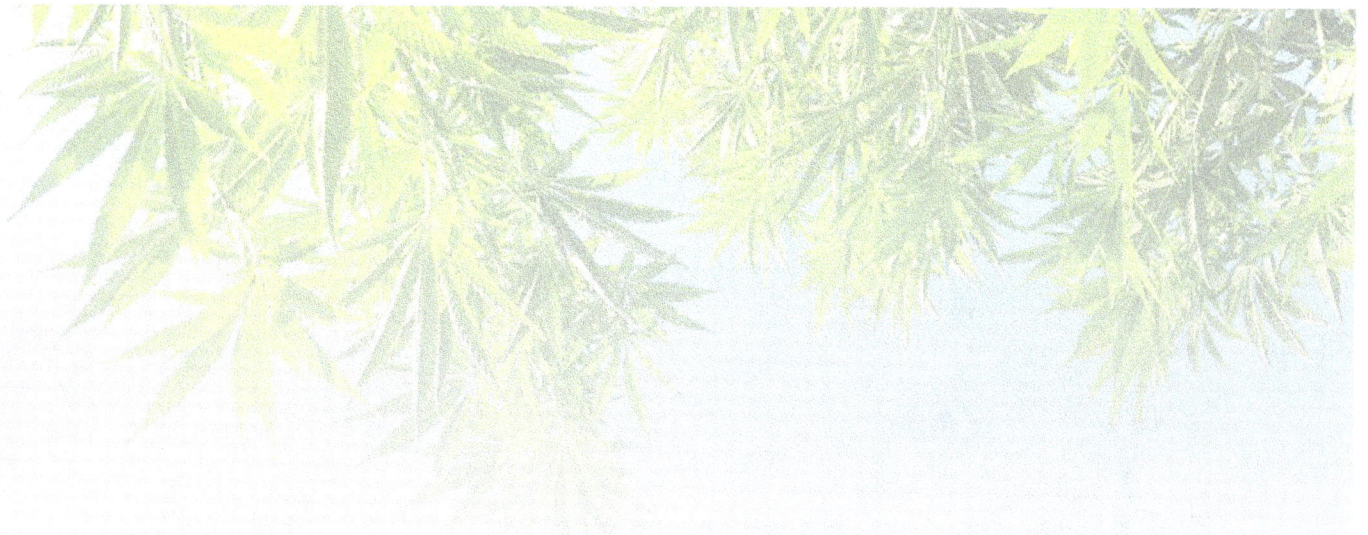

Humidity

You might think of humidity as something that occurs in the Deep South or tropical environments, but humidity can be found virtually everywhere – including your grow room. In general, about 40 to 80% relative humidity (rH) is ideal. Humidity is basically a measurement of the water in the air. Humidity is controlled through the use of fresh air (as stated above). Some growers even have an rH meter on hand to ensure the humidity stays within an ideal range. There are also expensive dehumidifiers that control humidity levels in a room, but they can be quite expensive. Unless you're planning on setting up a rather substantial operation, you can probably get by with a little fresh air once in a while.

Carbon Dioxide (CO2)

CO2 is another vital component that plants need to survive. CO2 isn't that great for humans, but plants like cannabis use CO2 as their air. It's basically the stuff that helps them breathe, but it is also vital for spurring and maintaining photosynthesis. If your grow room lacks enough CO2, it will likely become obvious. There are plenty of methods to increase CO2 in a room, but the best way is with a CO2 generator. These generators will keep a steady flow of CO2 coming into the room, which the plants will easily consume. There's almost no way to overfeed cannabis plants with CO2 unless you somehow go really overboard. For instance, if the grow room is unsafe for you to breathe, then you might need to tone it down a little. Otherwise, the amount of carbon dioxide in the room is directly proportional to how large the plant (and later the buds) will end up growing.

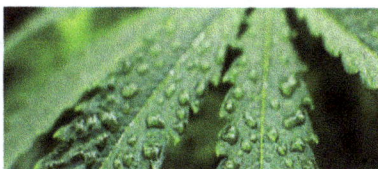

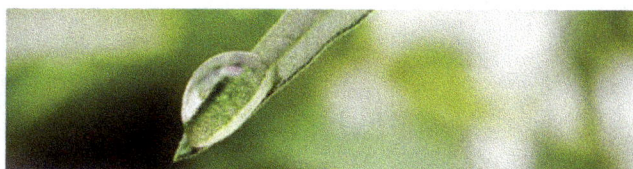

FLOWERING

Because you're growing indoors, when your plants begin to flower is almost wholly dependent on when you want the plants to flower. Of course, you want them to flower when the buds are at their highest potency. It's feasible to keep a marijuana plant in a vegetative state for up to 10 years, but those plants certainly won't be potent by the end of such a long lifespan. Before you induce flowering, make sure you know which plants are male and which ones are female.

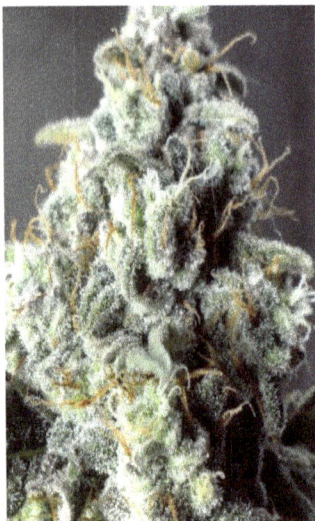

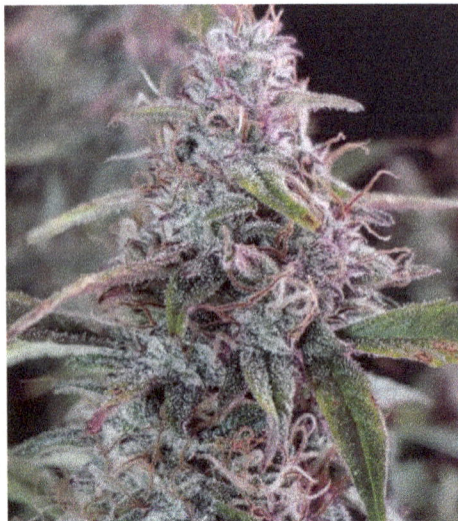

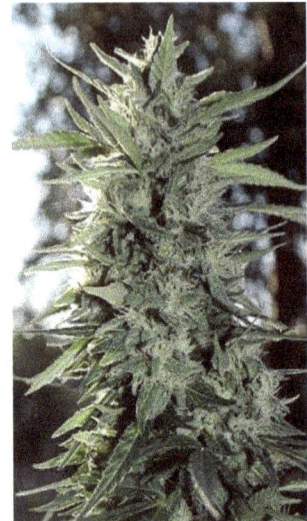

DETERMINING THE SEX

In general, marijuana plants start to "pre-flower" before you even manipulate them to flower. During this time, they will exhibit subtle signs of their sex. Male plants will generally start to pre-flower earlier than females (by around two weeks). You'll notice the male plants growing taller than the females. They also might develop sacs that resemble buds but aren't actually buds. The reason the male plants grow faster and taller than the female plants is so they can pollinate them. The pollen in the sacs (or false buds) will drop down onto the females to start the pollination process.

By contrast, the female plant will enter the pre-flowering stage by producing white, hairy growths at the nodes and on the top cola (the head). These are called pistils, and they are what attract the male pollen to the female plant.

There's really no surefire way to determine the sex of your plants until they start exhibiting these telltale signs. You can, however, take a cutting from one of the plants and plant it in an area separate from your garden. The cutting is basically a clone of its "mother" plant and will share the exact same genetic structure. You can then force the clone to flower, causing it to definitively start to show signs of its sex. Then, you can go back to your garden and label each plant that you do this for.

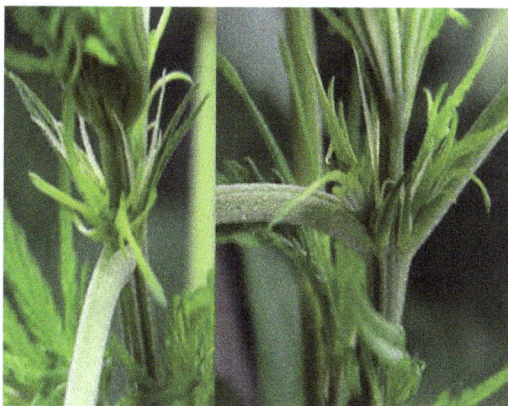

Female plant

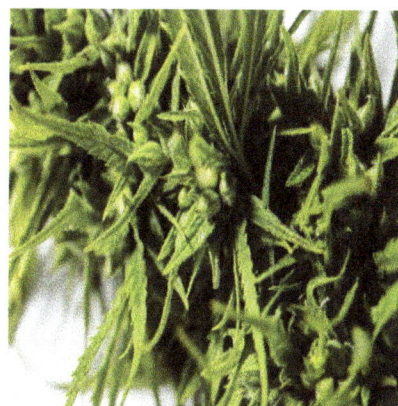

Male plant

Many growers want to determine the sex as soon as possible because the female plants will naturally produce a much better high. That's not to say that the males are useless, but you still want to distinguish between the two so that you know what you have. This is particularly true for growers who want "sinsemilla" buds. Sinsemilla literally means "without seed" in Spanish and, if the males are not allowed to pollinate the females, the plants will not produce any seeds. These seedless female plants are considerably more potent than their counterparts because they focus more attention on THC production and bud growth rather than on producing seeds. In fact, you can practically see the THC resin dripping off their buds.

Of course, you'll need to take out the male plants early to produce these types of buds. If you rely on your own garden for seeds for next year's harvest, then this probably wouldn't be a good idea. As mentioned before, buying seeds from a dealer or even a seed-bank is often a random grab bag. You don't know what the seeds will become, and receiving a full batch of males is not outside the realm of possibility. Letting your male plants pollinate the female plants will provide you with plenty of seeds, and you won't have to pay for them.

It is also possible to end up with hermaphroditic plants, which are basically just plants that have both sets of reproductive organs. Thus, they might exhibit early signs of both male and female plants. Stress can cause Hermaphrodite marijuana plants. Most growers also eliminate these plants from their crop even if they want to pollinate the females. While they are self-pollinating, they will only ever produce hermaphroditic plants, and they might even pollinate some non-hermaphroditic plants. It might seem like the best of both worlds, but your potency will be limited in these plants.It should also be noted that male plants aren't useless in terms of smoking either. They can still produce a little bit of a high and can also be used in culinary preparations. However, it's critical to take out the males if you want to grow sinsemilla marijuana. One male marijuana plant can pollinate hundreds of females.

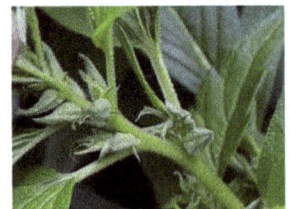

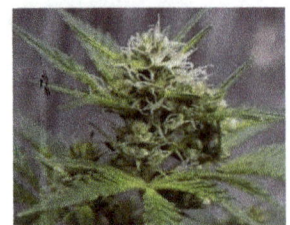

Hermaphrodite plants

How to Force Flowering

Now that you know how to check for the signs of male and female plants, the next step is getting them to flower properly. Just remember that, once you start flowering, it might be difficult to stop the males from pollinating the females if you haven't removed them. Even if you segregate the plants by their sex, the air still might carry some of the pollen to the female pistils. It's really a decision between whether you want hyper-potent buds for this year only or to keep growing your favorite strain without having to pay for new seeds. (Most personal growers will want to stick with the latter option because paying for your own seeds every year can be costly).

In any event, if you want to force flowering, all you have to do is put the plants on a 12-12 light regimen. That essentially means that you'll need to leave the lights on for only about 12 hours per day and turn them off for the remaining 12 hours.

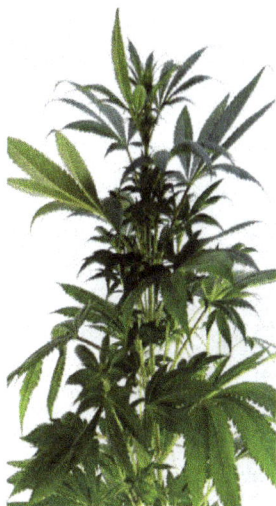

Flowering week 3   Flowering week 6   Flowering week 8

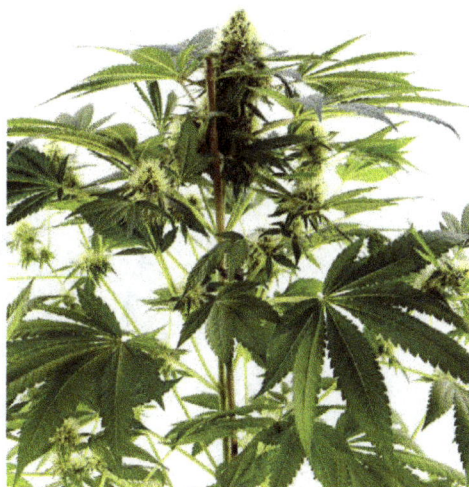

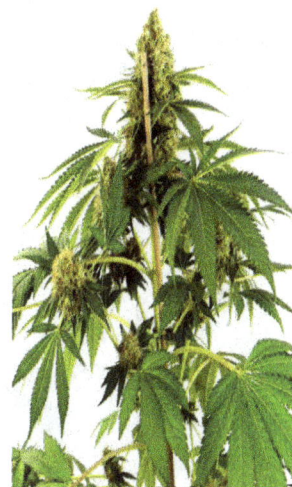

The room should be kept as dark as possible during the 12-hour dark period. Turning off the lights won't always do the trick, especially if there are other light sources nearby. In fact, even shining a flashlight on the plants for a few minutes at a time during the dark period can keep them in vegetative growth. If you have windows in your grow room, do your best to block them out, especially if the sun comes up before the 12-hour period is over. If your lights came equipped with a timer, then it's a good idea to set that so you don't have to worry about manually turning the lights on and off every 12 hours.

You'll notice that the female plants will start to grow larger as the flowering period progresses. They will grow more branches, buds, and flowers, and the plant will begin to produce more THC overall. The plants will take on a sort of cone shape that resembles a Christmas tree, and you might even start to smell a distinctive fruity or smoky aroma. Their pistils will change from their whitish color to a darker shade (generally brown, red, or orange); at that point, they should be ripe enough for picking. Even if you want to pollinate your female plants, you might consider removing the male plants post-pollination so that the females have more room to flourish.

The plants start to flower when the light and dark periods are both 12 hours long because they are genetically programmed to do so. If you plant outdoors (more on that later), you'll find that the plants will start to flower naturally when daylight begins to dwindle in the fall.

See here our High Yielding strains. I also created a High Yielding Mixpack to try 3 strains at the same time!

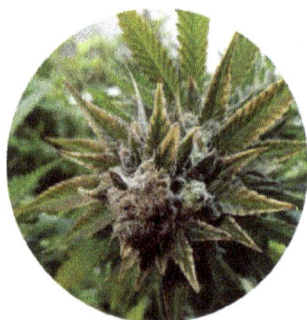

Northern Lights

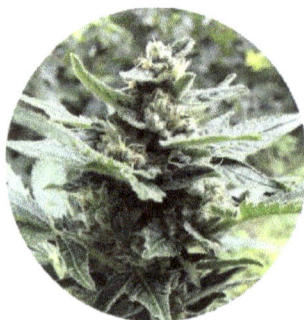

White Widow

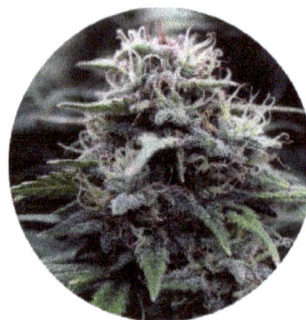

Big Bud

INDOOR PROBLEMS AND PESTS

For the most part, indoor growers won't have to worry about any diseases or pests plaguing their plants. But that doesn't mean it's entirely impossible. In general, microbial diseases are minimal because the microbes that affect plants usually don't exist in Europe or North America (where many of you are likely growing).

Nutrient issues occur, but those are from the plant receiving too many or too few nutrients. This can be remedied in a number of ways that are outlined in the "Indoor Vegetative Growth" section above.

Pests are really what you need to focus on preventing or eliminating if they make their way into your house. This is because, in nature, these pests would be mitigated by their natural predators, but in an enclosed system like the inside of your house, they won't have anything but you to stop them. Of course, the best option when it comes to these pests is always prevention. But some of the most insidious plant pests, like mites and whiteflies, are very difficult to detect. You can bring them in on your hands or clothes, or they might slip through cracks in your windows. It's also possible that the mites could have already been in your house to begin with. Many houseplants are resistant to these types of pests, but that doesn't mean that they aren't there; it just means that they don't hurt the houseplant.

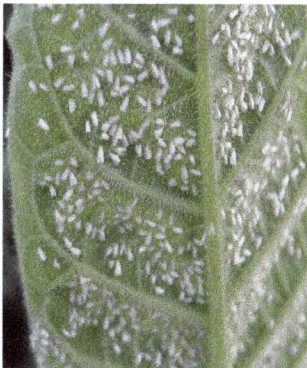
White flies

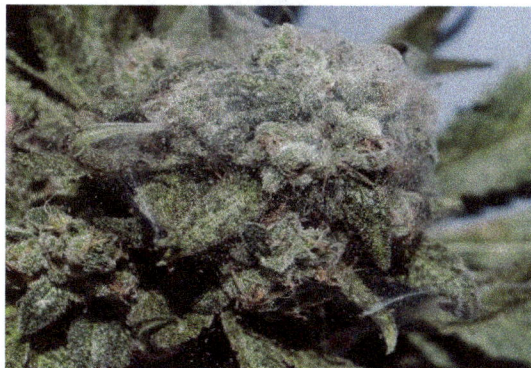
Spider mites

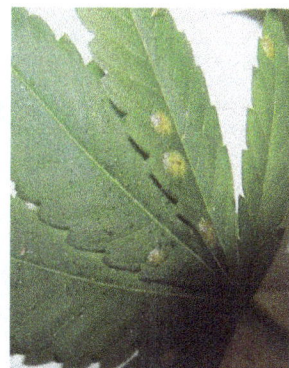
Mealybugs

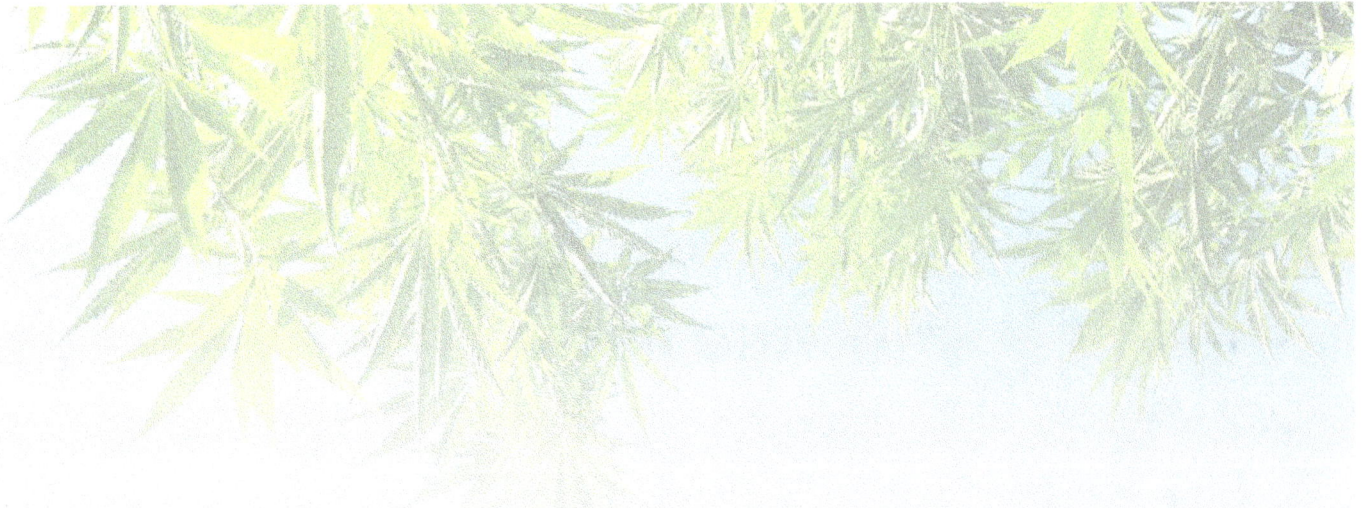

If you have a houseplant that's resistant to mites and other pests, it could already be infested with many of these creatures. You can test this out by placing a marijuana seedling in the pot with the other houseplant. If the seedling starts to show signs of drooping or a lack of vitality, or if the leaves start turning a whitish color, then you probably already have mites in your house.

Never use the same tools for your houseplants and your marijuana garden. If you have windows in the grow room, install a nylon mesh or wire screen to prevent pests from accessing your garden. Also, make sure that the soil you use is pasteurized and thoroughly sterilized so that it doesn't contain any larval eggs.

Pests can be devastating for your marijuana plants. If you suspect any intruders in your grow room, be sure to act immediately.

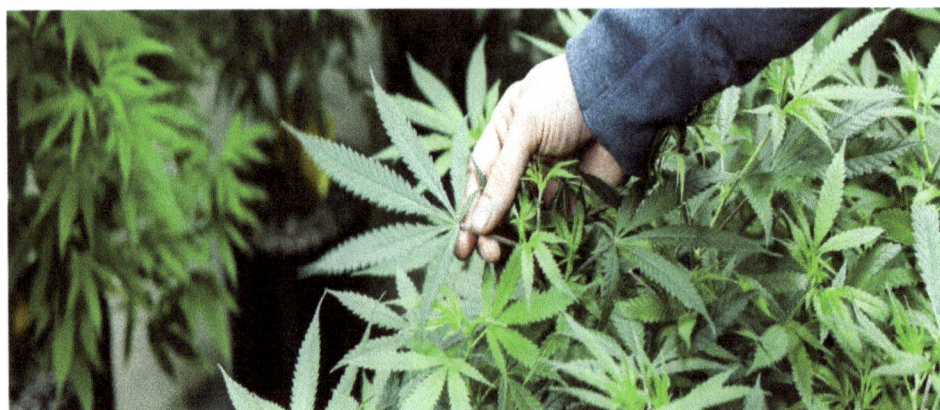

Eliminating Pests

If you still end up with an infestation of mites or whiteflies (or any other pests), then there are a few things you can do to get rid of them. Insecticides will work, of course, but many people don't want to harm their plants with the chemicals they contain. If the plants are otherwise healthy but you can see some significant deterioration of the leaves, then you might want to begin force flowering right away. If the pests only infected a few plants or a few leaves, you can simply remove the infected sections. Plants that are already in the flowering stage will likely survive any pests without a problem.

If the problem still persists, you might want to think about using an insecticide. Sprays that include things like pyrethrum, rotenone, and malathion are generally considered safe when used correctly. Just remember that you don't have to spray an entire canister on your plants to get the job done. Remove any affected leaves before spraying, and don't use any insecticide during flowering. The best part about these varieties of insecticides is that they degrade into safe chemical compounds, such as CO_2 or water, when they stop working. There are also natural solutions that you can make, but they aren't as effective.

Protect your plants from diseases and harmful pests with the Plant Protector and make sure you don't have to worry about a thing but growing big strong buds!

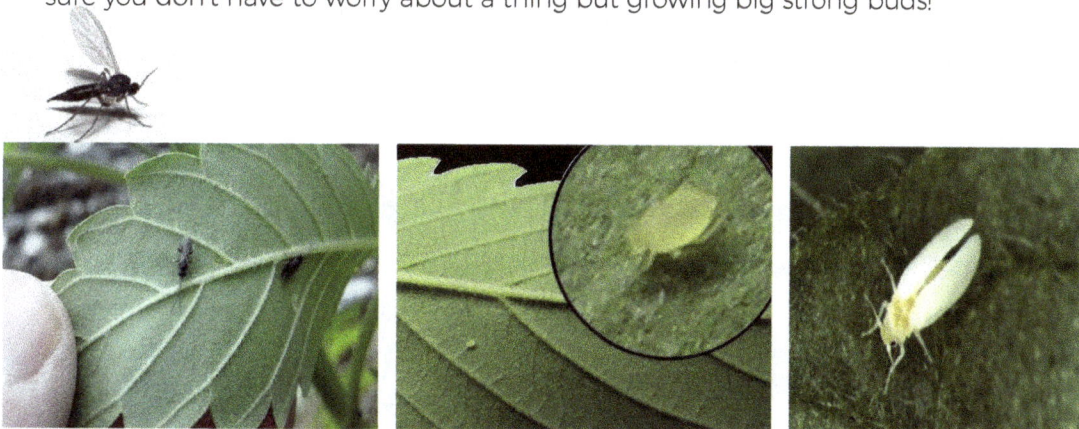

A Few Notes about Security

Although most people grow indoors to avoid any security issues, there are still some problems that can occur if you're not careful. In many jurisdictions, growing marijuana is still clearly illegal, and, if someone thinks there's reason to suspect that you are growing, you could wind up behind bars (or at least paying a hefty fine).

The first rule about growing marijuana is to not talk about growing marijuana too much. Even if you feel like you're friendly with your neighbor or your bank teller or an acquaintance, they might not be friendly with the practice of growing marijuana.

If you have a window in your grow room, concealing the marijuana plants won't be that easy unless your window isn't visible to your neighbors or anyone else from the outside. Also, if you leave the grow lights on at night, it might lead someone to suspect that something illicit is going on. To avoid that, you can buy a blackout curtain that you leave pulled down for most of the time you spend growing marijuana. A blackout curtain will also help make the flowering period easier because it ensures that no outside light will leak in.

Sometimes your marijuana plants will give off a distinct smell that anyone will recognize as cannabis. It might be a relatively strong smell wafting out of any open windows. The scent might make your neighbors suspicious, particularly if they are not proponents of growing cannabis. In this case, you might need to keep your window firmly closed and install fans in the grow room (instead of opening the windows) to circulate the air.

OUTDOOR GROWING

Many growers prefer to grow their marijuana seeds outdoors because of the possibility of a better smoke, plus there is undoubtedly nothing more natural than growing your plants outside. Most of the environmental factors outlined above are provided to the plant via natural resources, saving you from having to create them. While indoor growing gives you a lot of control, outdoor growing lets the plants flourish to their fullest capacity.

The main problem with outdoor growing, however, is that the plants are visible to anyone who happens to have prying eyes. If you live in a residential neighborhood, you might be able to get away with growing your plants in your backyard, but you'll likely need to be somewhat paranoid about keeping the operation under wraps. Even then, you could still be caught, and the penalties for that are potentially severe.

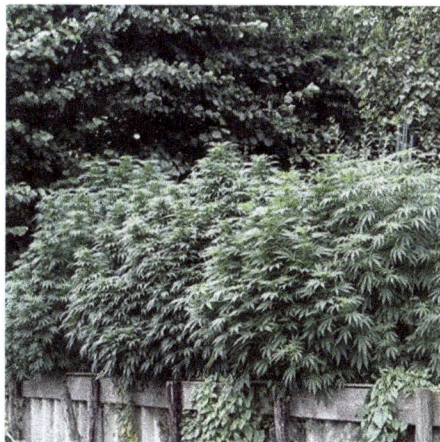

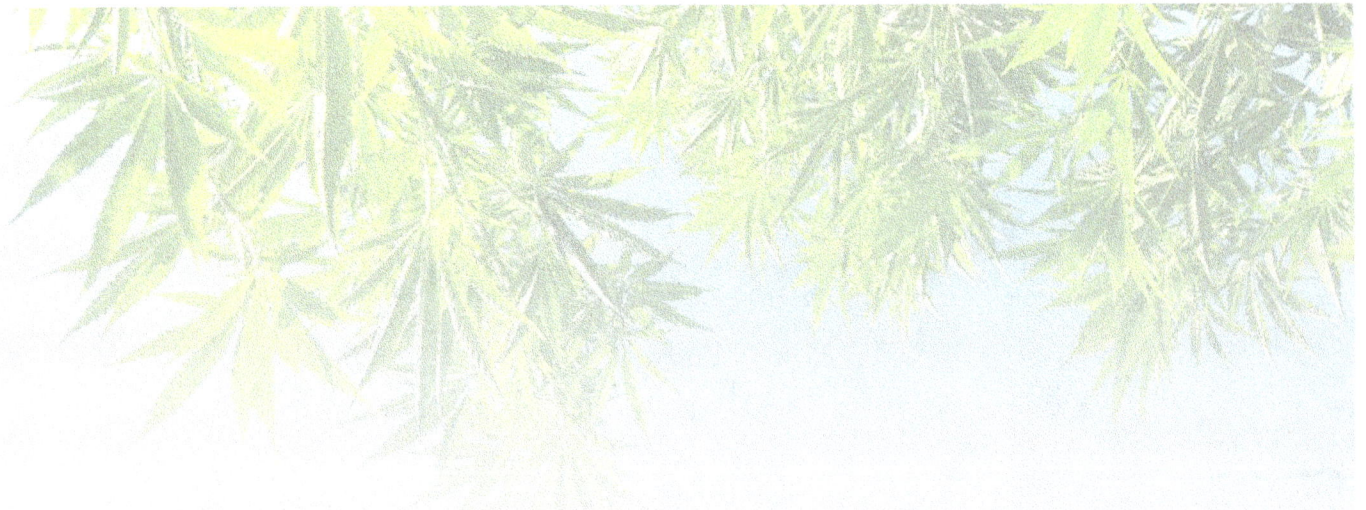

If you live in a secluded or wooded area and you own a lot of land, then it might be a little easier to grow your own smoke on your personal property. For instance, if you live on ranchland (or you have access to a friend's ranchland), then you might be able to grow outdoors with minimal interference. This is really the ideal way to go about it because you can inspect the plants whenever you want without the fear of being caught. You can also avoid the hassle of having to deal with thieves looking to score your homemade bud.

Unfortunately, many people don't have access to secluded private land that wouldn't arouse suspicion from law enforcement or other individuals. Thus, if they want the best bud, they will have to employ a system known as "guerrilla farming." This means that you'll have to go to public lands that are somewhat off the beaten path to grow your garden. There are obvious dangers to doing this because anyone could happen to come across your garden and alert the proper authorities. It's also not uncommon for law enforcement to survey many public lands using helicopters or slow-flying planes. The police are equipped with infrared devices that can point out any irregularities in foliage. If the spot you planted your garden is in an open space, the plants will likely be clearly visible to anyone flying by. But, if you plant underneath some dense foliage, they might just blend in with the rest of the trees and shrubs in the area.

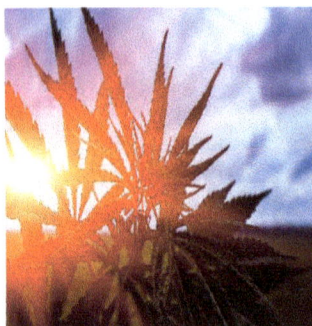

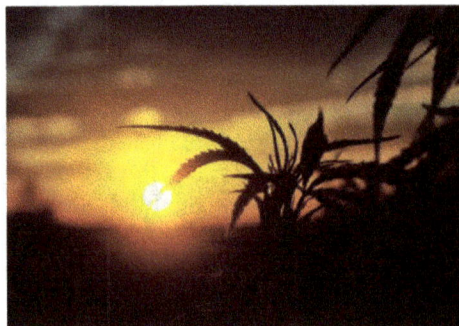

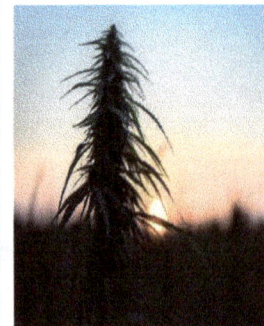

Soil

Regardless of where you're growing outside, good soil is imperative. But not every kind of dirt will be ideal for growing marijuana. It's always a good idea to test the ground soil that you're planning to grow in before actually using it. This is to ensure that it won't be too alkaline or acidic when the plants start extending their roots even deeper into the ground. If the pH balance is too much in either direction then you might want to consider a new location or infuse the soil with some nutrients and fertilizers.

Many growers like to use composted material as a natural fertilizer. Anything that once was organic can be used as compost. This means that you can gather leaves, banana peels, and even dog droppings, and in a few months you'll have a nice, nutrient-rich fertilizer. Obviously, you can't just take the leaves or shrubs or banana peels and use them as a fertilizer if they haven't yet decayed. But virtually any decayed organic material works as a cheap fertilizer. If you want to get the pH to an acceptable level, use some of the techniques outlined in the "Soil Control" section above.

You can also buy fertilizers. A fertilizer with an NPK ratio of around 5:1:1 (just like before) will be the best option. Any fertilizer that has more nitrogen than the other two nutrients will be ideal for most of the plant's life, up until flowering (when more phosphorus is ideal.) Of course, if guerrilla farming is your preferred method of growing, then you won't really have these options at your disposal. In fact, unless you have a definitive location picked out months ahead of time, you won't really have the option of creating a more workable soil. You'll just have to go with what you can find, as hiking in your own fertilizer could make it exceedingly obvious that you're growing something out there.

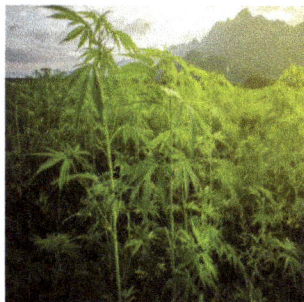

Plant in green areas   Make your own container   Corn and marijuana need the same soil

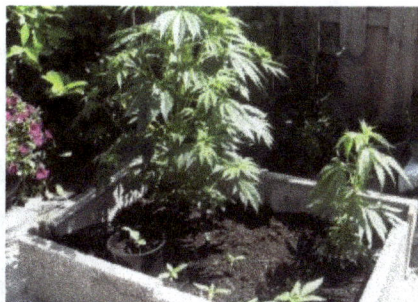

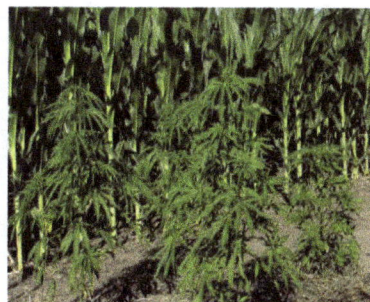

Sowing the Seeds

Many growers like to start out their seeds in rows created in the soil. You don't really need to bury the seeds very deep in the soil. In fact, some growers simply scatter their seeds on top of the soil to get them to germinate. This random seeding is called broadcast seeding.

A more effective way to sow your seeds is by using hills or mounds. For this method, the seeds go on top of the small mounds of soil. With this technique, you can plant outdoors even when the ground is somewhat wet. This is because the water is naturally going to drain off of the mound so the seed (and, later, the plant) won't be inundated. In either the hill or row option, try to ensure that the seeds have adequate soil coverage so that they can stay moist.

Most guerilla farmers use broadcast seeding to limit any suspicion and because it's a lot easier. If you spend hours building rows or mounds, there is a strong likelihood that someone could happen to notice you. It's also rare to see any uniformity in nature. If your plants are ordered in perfect rows, or they are all sitting atop a small mound of some kind, then any passersby (whether on the ground or in the air) is probably going to take notice of the anomaly. Scattering the seeds around definitely gives the area a look of complete arbitrariness, the way nature might have intended. The plants will blend in with all of the other scattered trees and/or shrubs and won't be easily noticed by anyone else. Here you can see sowing in rows and broadcast seeding.

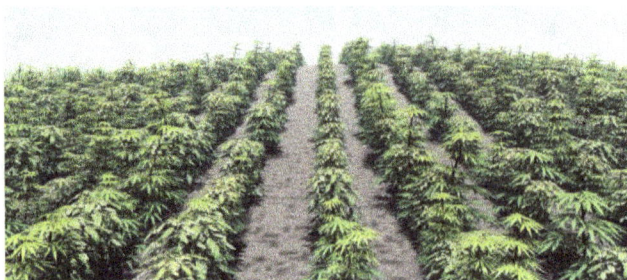

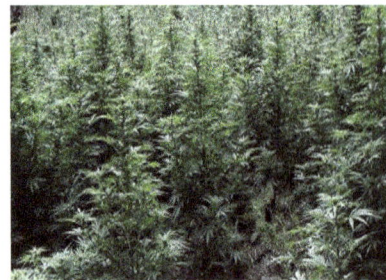

Unfortunately, broadcast seeding isn't the best way to ensure that your plants will germinate. If you place a layer of soil over your seeds and gently press them down into the soil with your foot, there's a better chance that the seeds will germinate. Many seeds, however, will never germinate or will simply die after becoming seedlings if you try to grow in this fashion. That's why using a large amount of seeds for broadcast seeding is crucial so that you are at least guaranteed some growth by the time they start germinating.

Germination

Just like with indoor germination, outdoor seeds require moisture to germinate properly. Adding too much water can be detrimental, but as long as the seeds are surrounded by at least some moisture they should start to germinate. Of course, this is easier if you built mounds or rows for the seeds, as they naturally maintain moisture.

Sometimes, the conditions outside are not conducive to germination or the subsequent seedling stage. If you live in an area where the temperatures remain relatively low well into spring then you may need to germinate the seeds indoors. To do this, just follow the instructions laid out in the indoor growing section on germination above. Then you can transplant the seedlings when the weather starts to improve.

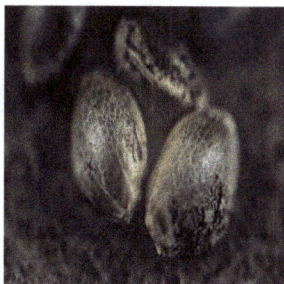

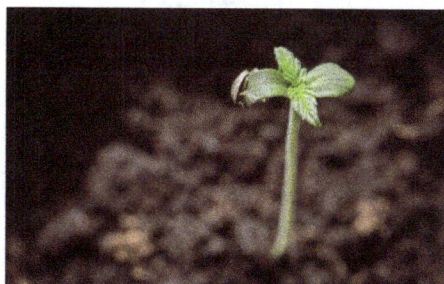

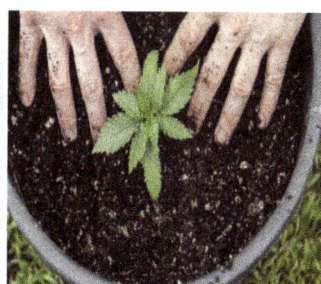

Again, transplanting to a secluded location on public land is pointless at best and dangerous at worst. There's a strong likelihood that the plants won't survive the transplant because of all the stress they would be put under. There is also a strong likelihood that you could be caught because it would probably take more than one trip to get all of your plants in the right position. The whole germination process is difficult for guerrilla farmers, especially if there isn't a reliable source of water nearby. Hauling in your own water is challenging, but the soil needs to be moist for the seeds to germinate so it may be vital.

Weeding

As your plants start to germinate, it's essential to keep the area free of weeds. Avoid using any weed killers like Round-Up that might also affect your marijuana plants. Weeds are dangerous because they will end up taking a lot of the water and nutrients meant for your plants if you don't stamp them out quickly. The best way to get rid of weeds is by merely pulling them out by hand. Trying to kill them with any chemicals will only be bad for the plants that you are trying to grow to be big and strong. Naturally, before planting in an area you should pull out any weeds that happen to be there.

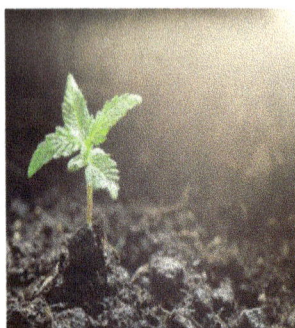

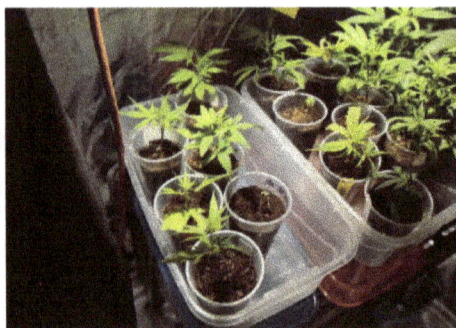

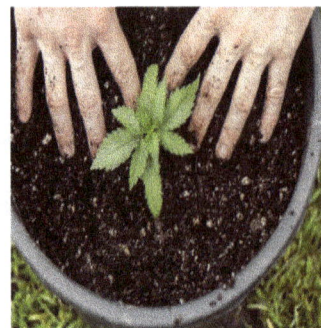

Light

The benefit of being in the great outdoors is that you don't really need to worry about light too much. The sun will provide all the light a plant could need and much more. There is no way to duplicate the sun's intensity, and it's just a better light source than anything you could produce artificially.

If you transplant your plants from indoor artificial light to outdoor sunlight, however, they could be shocked by the intensity. This would certainly not be an ideal way to start your outdoor growing experience as you might see the plants lose vigor and ultimately die. If you sowed the seeds outdoors in the bright sunlight, your plants will already be acclimated to the sun for the rest of their lives. However, when transplanting from indoors to outdoors, you have to ease them into it. At first, place the plants in a location that has shade for part of the day to ensure that the sun's rays hit them directly but for a shorter period of time. This is assuming you will leave them in portable pots rather than planting them straight into the ground. As they start to get used to the sun's rays, gradually move them more into the direct sunlight until they are receiving light all day. It shouldn't take more than 7 or 10 days to get the plants acclimated to the sunlight.

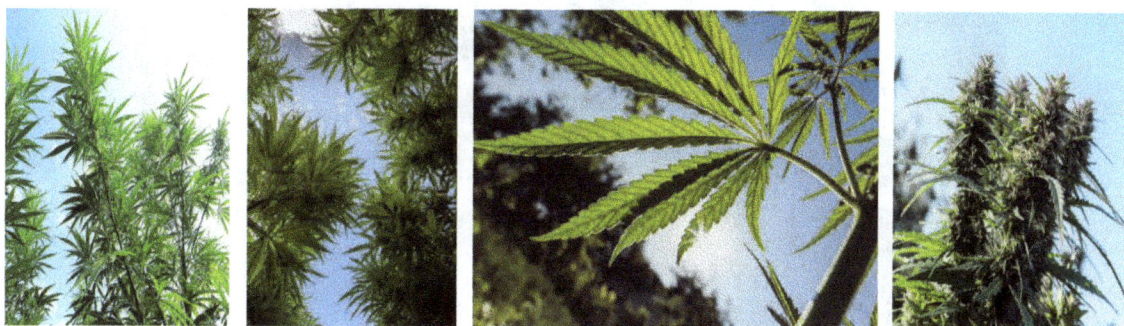

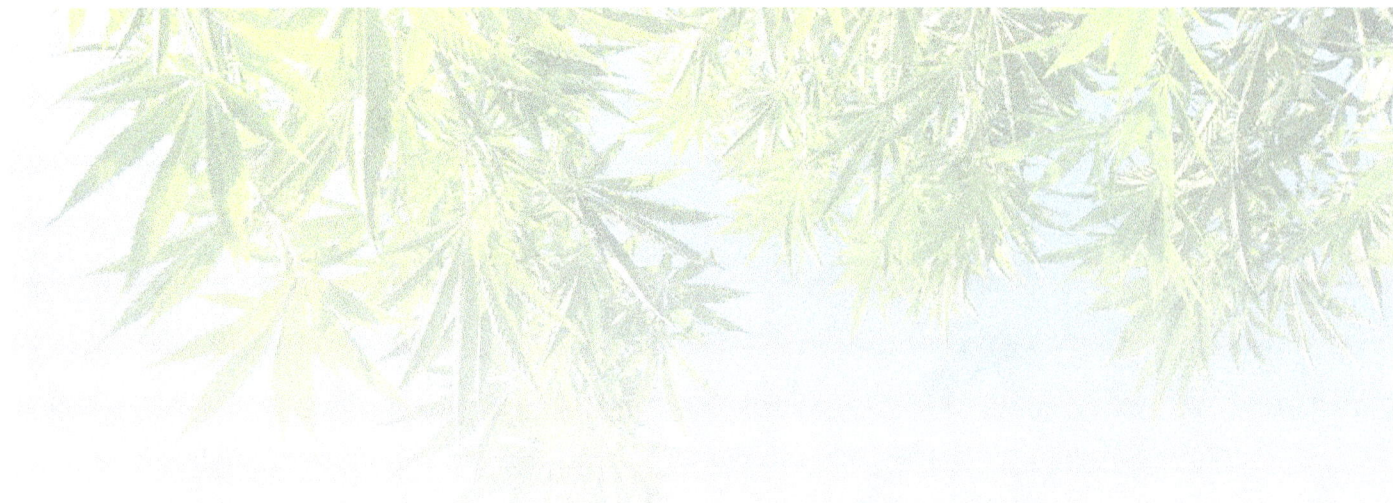

Light can also be a problem if something is blocking it from getting to your plants. If you live in a cloudy area, for instance, the plants might not be receiving enough direct light from the sun. You may have to bring the plants indoors at night and put them under some lamps, so they get a full dose of light for the day.

If you are guerrilla farming in a forested area, your plants might be at risk of having the light blocked out by taller trees in the area. Although the trees provide security and cover from any potential onlookers, they may also limit the amount of light that your plants receive. It will be difficult to transplant them once they are in the ground so you may just have to deal with the limited amount of light.

Some growers utilize the landscape to receive the most light. When planting on the slope of a mountain, make sure that you plant on the south side (if you're in the Northern Hemisphere). This is because the sun will go from east to west, but it will be in the southern half of the sky. If the plants are on the southern slope of the mountain, they will receive the most sunlight possible throughout the day.

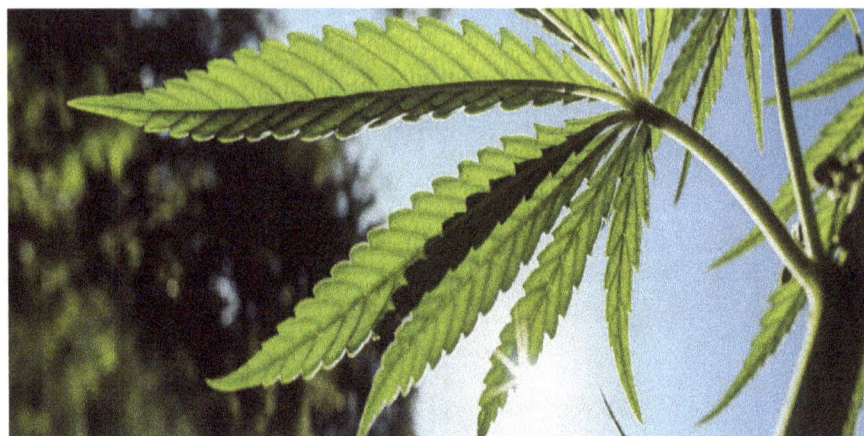

Watering

Watering your outdoor plants can be kind of tricky, especially if they are located in a relatively dry and arid place. If your plants aren't close to a hose then you'll have to devise a plan to get your plants as much water as possible. Obviously, early on, the plants won't need a lot in the way of H_2O but, as they enter into vegetative growth and start to get much larger, they will need more water. Large adult plants can consume up to a gallon of water per day. This doesn't mean that you'll have to water the plants with a gallon of water every day because the soil should retain some of the water from previous waterings (or even from rain).

If your plants are on private land that you have access to, there is no shortage of unique techniques that you can use to get water to your plants. For instance, you can fill buckets up with water and transport them by truck to the grow site. Try to avoid oversaturating your plants with water by dumping too much water on a single one.

Other growers set up a drip method of watering with something like a squeeze bottle that has a permanent drip. This technique allows the growers to avoid having to water the plants every day while still keeping the soil moist on a continuous basis. Although it is gradual by nature, the drip method keeps the plants relatively healthy and doesn't flood them with too much water.

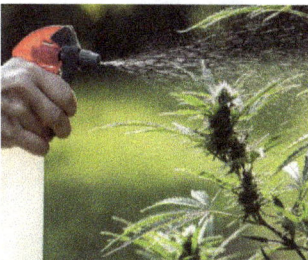

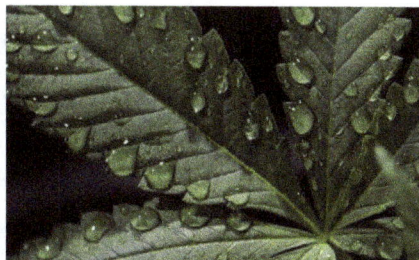

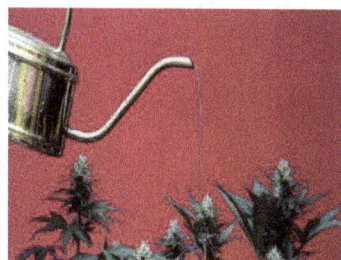

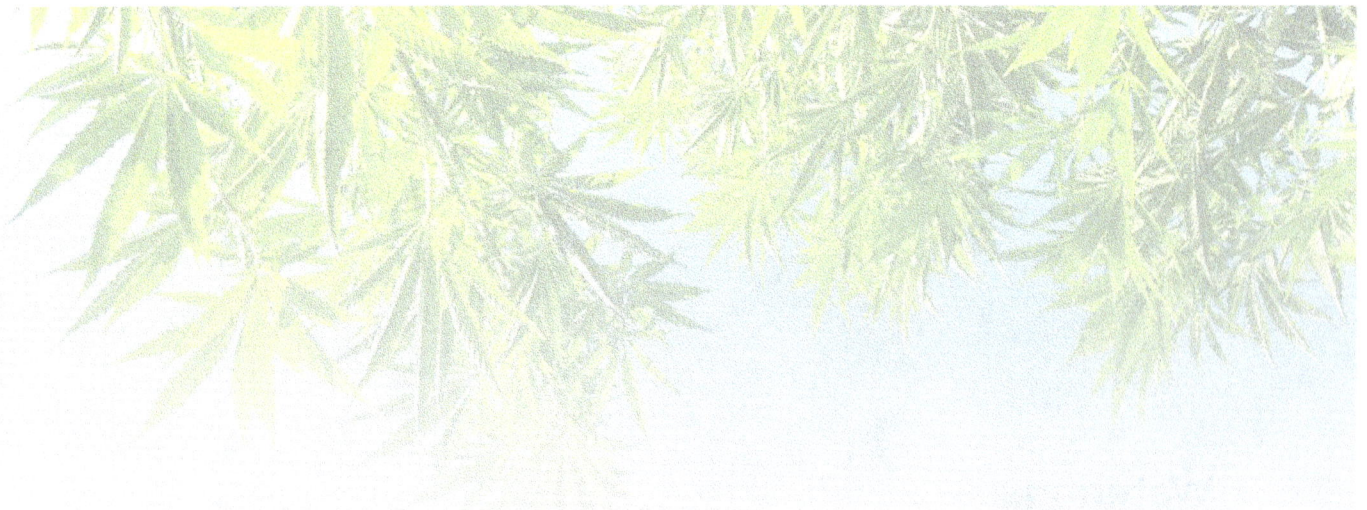

Of course, you might live in an area where cannabis can grow naturally without the use of any extra water on your end. This is ideal for guerrilla farmers who likely won't be able to check on their plants on a daily basis. If you are a guerrilla farmer and you live in an area where the weather is often hot and dry, then you might need to keep a firm watch on the plants. Hauling in your own water will be challenging on a number of levels, and it's better if you can find a nearby lake or stream that can provide water for you naturally.

If your plants are underwatered they will likely start wilting, but be aware that plants will naturally start wilting in the summer as a response to the heat of the sun. The best way to check if your plants are getting enough water is to dig about 6 inches into the soil, making sure not to cut any major roots on the way down. If the soil there is still cool and moist, the plants should be fine. Many types of soil are adept at holding water for long periods of time so that there is essentially a reservoir of water stored within it.

If at all possible, you might want to water your plants with a nutrient solution about once every couple of weeks. As long as the nutrient solution has a higher concentration of nitrogen than phosphorus and potassium, it will be good for vegetative growth. For flowering, use a solution that is higher in phosphorus than either of the other two nutrients. This should be done when you water the plants.

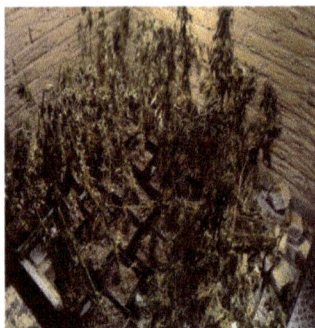

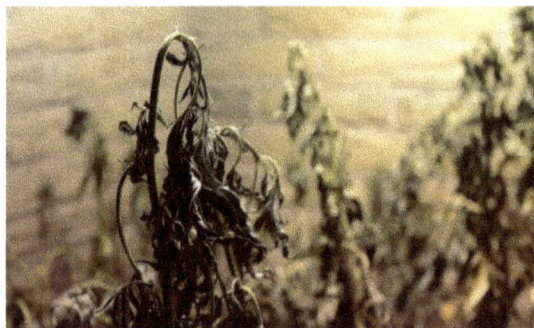

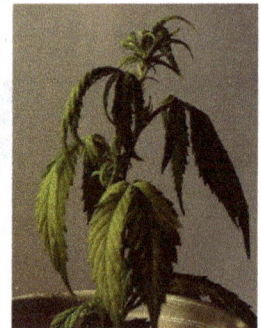

Underwatered marijuana plants

Temperature, Weather, and Air

Obviously, temperature is one of the major issues when growing outdoors. There's not a lot you can do to keep your plants warm enough or cool enough if there are weather problems. If your plants are still in pots, then you can move them indoors to avoid any excessive cold at night. When the temperature is particularly hot outside, the roots can start to sort of "boil" in the soil. Keeping them cool with extra water will help ensure that the plants don't begin to lose vigor.

Of course, being outdoors leaves your plants open for a large variety of other weather problems. Wind, rain, and snow (depending on where you live and when you plant) can all be problems that will hurt your plants. For the most part, high winds won't have much effect on healthy cannabis plants. They generally grow firm stalks that won't need any exterior support to stay standing. Indeed, most high winds will cause some tiny cracks in the plants' stalks, but, if they are healthy, they will heal themselves quite easily.

If the plants are suffering from nutrient deficiencies, however, they may have a hard time recuperating. This is also true if they are top heavy and therefore susceptible to more angled bends of the stalk. In this case, you might think about staking the plants so that they don't experience any irreparable damage. If you know a storm is coming, it's best to find your weakest plants and make sure they have some exterior support to mitigate the damage that the storm might cause.

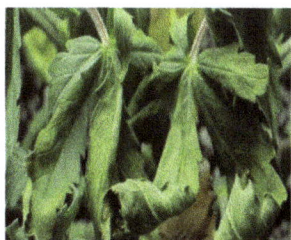

Not enough rain

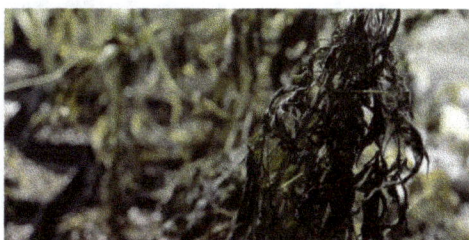

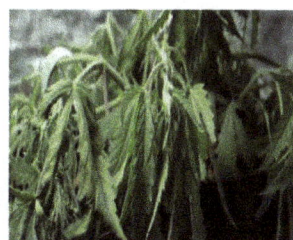

Too much rain, bad drainage

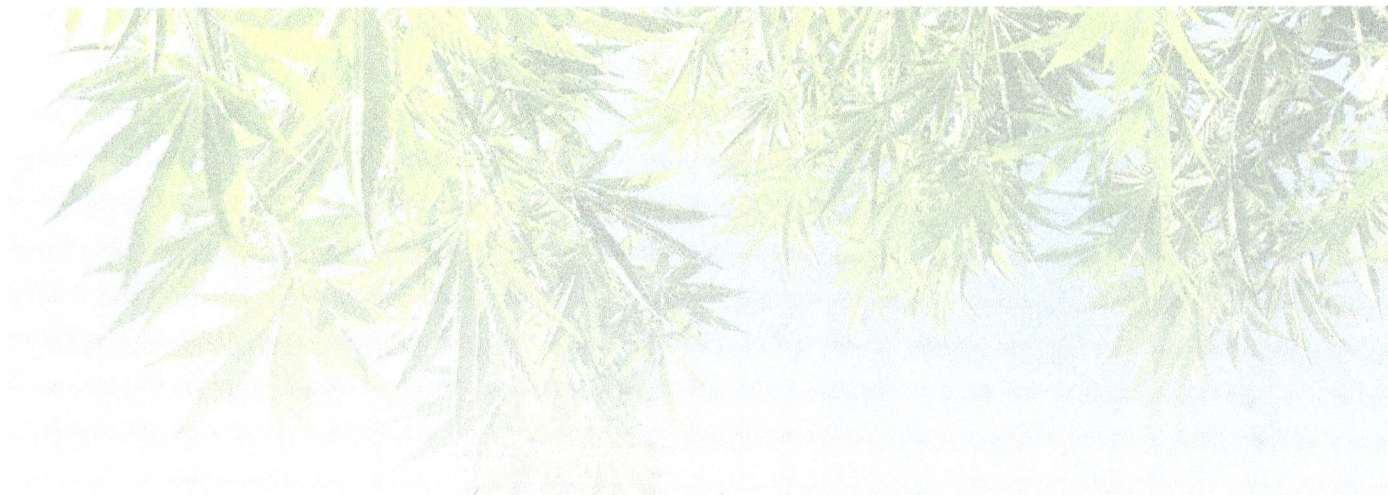

To do this, simply place a stake about six inches from the base of the plant, and then tie the plant and the stake together with wire twists or string.

For guerrilla farmers, it's a good idea to avoid planting in areas that are prone to mudslides. But not every slope is going to be an obvious mudslide area. A good indication that an area won't be adequate for your plants is if there aren't any other small plants growing there. If all you see is sturdy trees or shrubs, then the slope likely does not support small vegetation. Not paying attention to these signs could wipe out your entire crop during one freak summer storm.

In terms of the air quality that your plants will experience, there's nothing better than the great outdoors. Your plants will get all the fresh air they need and plenty of CO_2 to stay healthy.

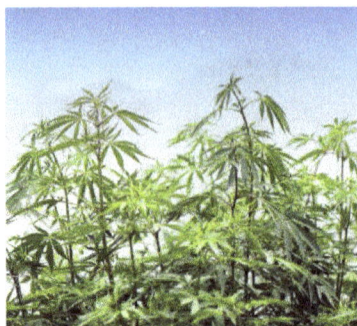

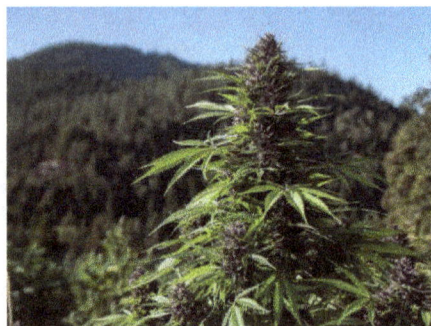

Outdoor Flowering

For the most part, flowering outdoors will require no input from the grower. Most plants will start adjusting to the changes in the daylight hours and begin the flowering process on their own. The days will naturally start to get shorter, which will trigger the plants into flowering organically.

For some growers, however, this will not be the ideal circumstance. Sometimes you don't want the plants to enter flowering, and sometimes you want them to enter it earlier. For instance, if the weather is still nice and you want to eke out all the vegetative growth you can in your plants, you'll want to delay flowering as long as possible. By that same token, if you know that the weather will soon become exceptionally cold or at least too cold for the plants to survive, then try to make sure that they start flowering sooner than they naturally would.

For growers that have access to their plants, both of these options are possible. If you want to delay the onset of flowering, it merely takes a little light during the night. You can accomplish this with a highpowered flashlight shining on the plants once every couple of hours or so for about 10 minutes during the night. This will adequately mess with the plants' natural inclination to start flowering and they will stay in vegetative growth for the time being.

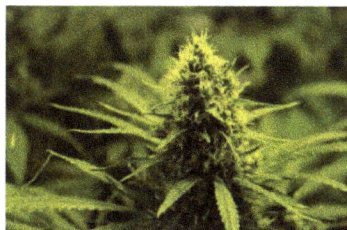

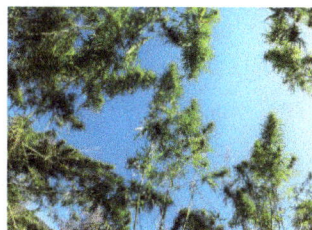

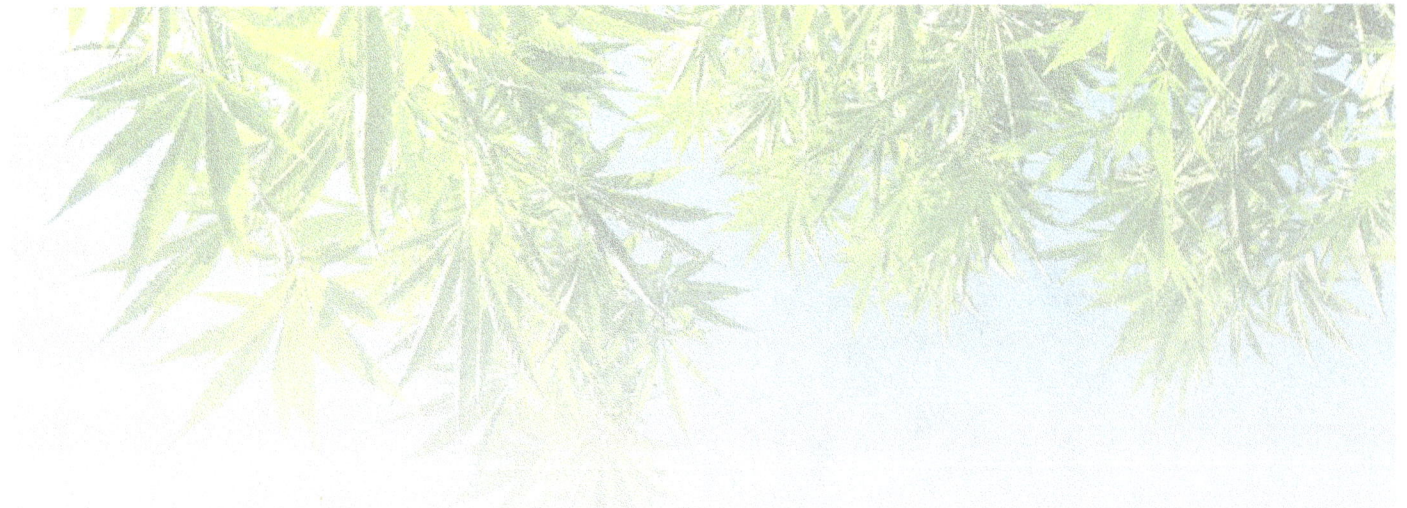

Obviously, if the weather starts to get cold early where you live, try to ensure that your plants start flowering as soon as possible. But outdoor plants offer certain challenges to this goal. If the light to darkness period isn't yet 12 hours to 12 hours then you'll need to make that happen on your own. Using a polyethylene sheet will help block out any sunrise or sunset light so that you can get the required 12 hours of darkness. For instance, if you know that your area is going to get exactly 13 hours of sunlight during the day and that sunset is at 7 PM, then place the sheet over the plants at 6 PM and remove it at 6 AM when the sun rises. After doing this for about 1 to 2 weeks, the plants should start to flower, and you can begin harvesting.

When it comes to manipulating the flowering period, guerrilla farmers are kind of out of luck. They will be at the mercy of the local weather in the area and won't have a lot of say in the matter. Just trust that nature will work its magic and find a way to give you some excellent smoke.

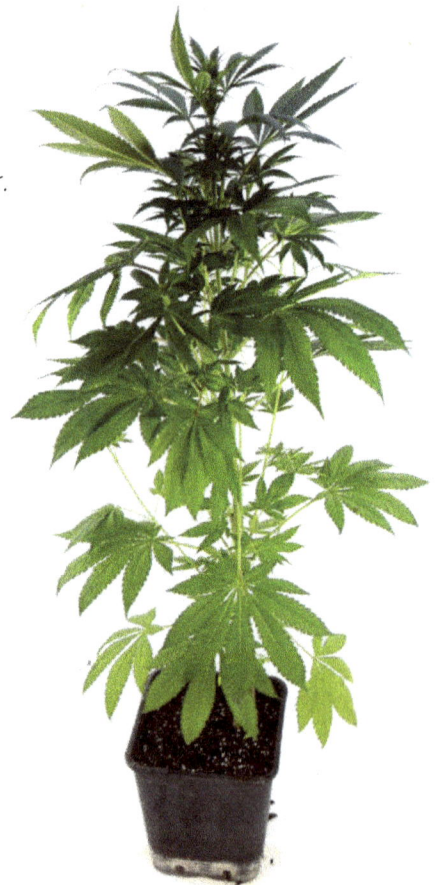

PESTS, PREDATORS AND OTHER PROBLEMS

You might expect outdoor plants to fare much worse than plants grown indoors when it comes to pests. That's true, but because the ecosystem is often self-regulating, there are many tricks to get rid of unwelcome visitors. For instance, even if a few bugs start munching on the leaves of your cannabis plants, it's likely that they will be held in check by any of their natural predators. Spider mites, aphids, whiteflies, and mealybugs are all common pests that many growers have to deal with both indoors and out. The plants are in the most danger when they are young and not well-developed. A single meal by a group of mites during a plant's seedling stage could cause some irreparable damage.

As the plant ages, however, it will start becoming less susceptible to insect damage. This is mainly because these insects will be taken care of by natural predators before the plant incurs much damage. If pests are a problem, there are a few options you can try to chase them away from your plants.

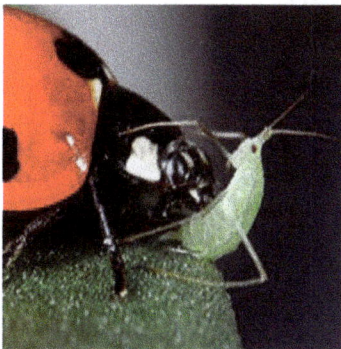

Ladybugs

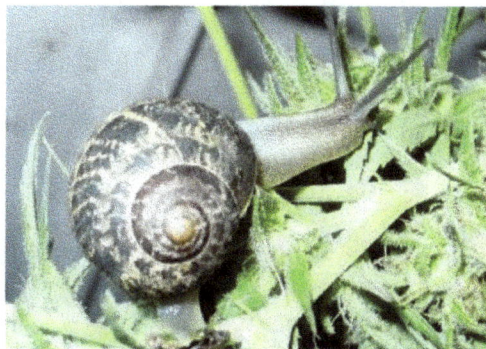

Snail

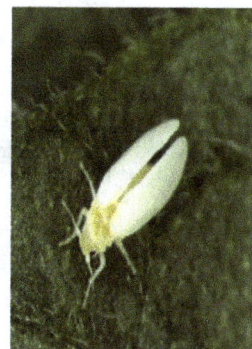

White flies

COMPANION PLANTING

Although the THC that marijuana produces is supposed to act as a natural repellent, it is sometimes not very helpful for getting rid of certain insects. Many outdoor growers have taken to planting companion plants that work to repel pests. In general, you must plant the companion plants near the actual marijuana plants.

The most effective repellent plants are those that have strong scents like herbs, spices, and mint. Garlic cloves are probably the best repellents because they ensure that a wide range of pests stay away from your garden. Aphids, spider mites, potato bugs, many types of beetles, and a wide range of other pests will be repelled by garlic cloves. Even rabbits and some deer will be put off by the scent that garlic cloves produce.

Mint is particularly effective at controlling flea beetles if you've got an unusually large infestation of them. They also repel a wide variety of other insects and even mice. Geraniums and marigolds can also be interspersed throughout your garden to provide an even larger range of protection. Geraniums can even be placed outside in pots so that you don't have to go through the hassle of actually planting them in the soil. Marigolds are some of the fastest growing flowers, and they will produce a strong scent within a few days.

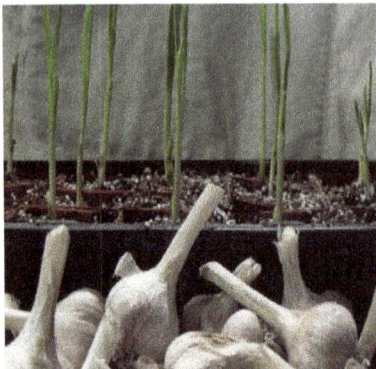

Garlic

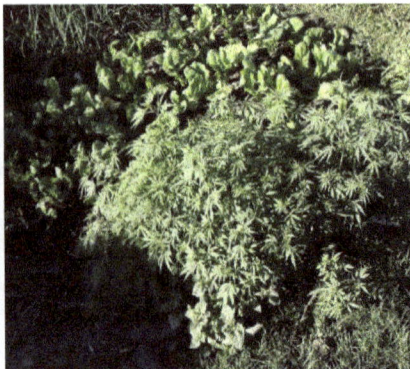

Other plants as camouflage

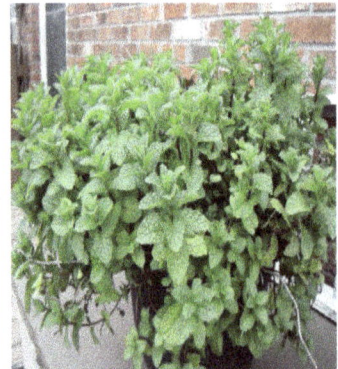

Mint

NATURAL PREDATORS

It's also possible to purchase the natural predators of these pests and place them in your garden. Other insects, such as ladybugs, have no interest in eating a marijuana plant, but they do have quite an appetite for aphids and insect eggs. Both praying mantises and lacewings also provide you with a natural way to rid yourself of any unwanted pests. All of these are sold commercially.

Several birds, including blue jays, robins, martins, chickadees, and others, are adept predators when it comes to killing off marijuanaloving pests. To attract these birds, some growers have installed birdhouses, feeders, and pools of water. It's also not a bad idea to let a few chickens, ducks, or geese run through the garden every once in a while as the plants grow larger. These birds will take out many pests along with a number of different weeds -- and you won't have to do any work. Other insect predators include frogs, toads, snakes, turtles, and lizards, which should all be encouraged to take up residence in your garden.

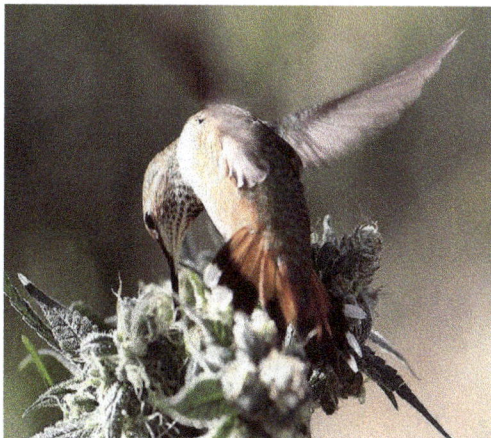

Birds eat insects

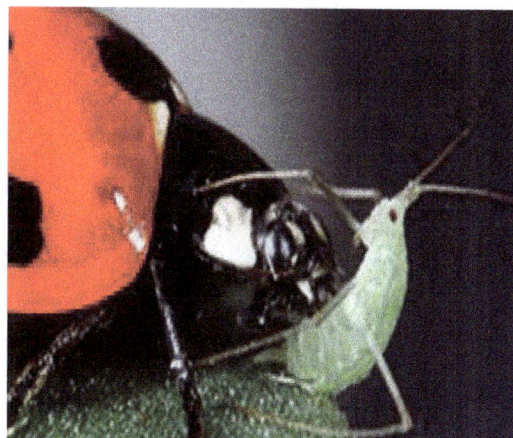

Ladybugs eat mites

OTHER REPELLENT METHODS

Many gardeners employ the use of some ingenious homemade sprays or other solutions that are remarkably effective. It's possible to use a concoction composed of liquid garlic extract and regular soap. You can also add cayenne peppers, onions, or almost anything else that is safe for the marijuana plant and also pungent enough to repel many different kinds of pests.

If you really want a cheap solution, you can literally just stomp on the bugs or squeeze them to death. It's best to do this in the early morning when the bugs are moving much slower in general. If anything, it gives you something to do before you head off to work or do whatever else you had planned for the day.

Many growers like to place barriers around their garden. This is particularly effective for guerrilla growers because it's hard to notice and doesn't take a lot of time to prepare. To do this, create a barrier about 6 feet away from the plant using powdered potash (wood ash). You can even sprinkle some of the wood ash onto the leaves to keep flying bugs at bay as well.

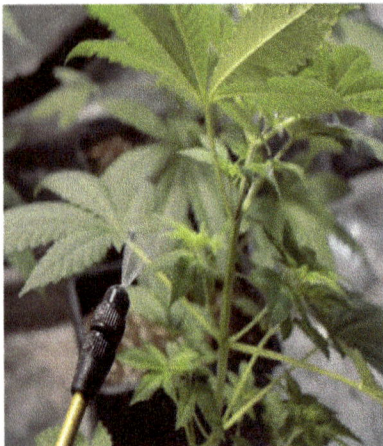

Homemade spray

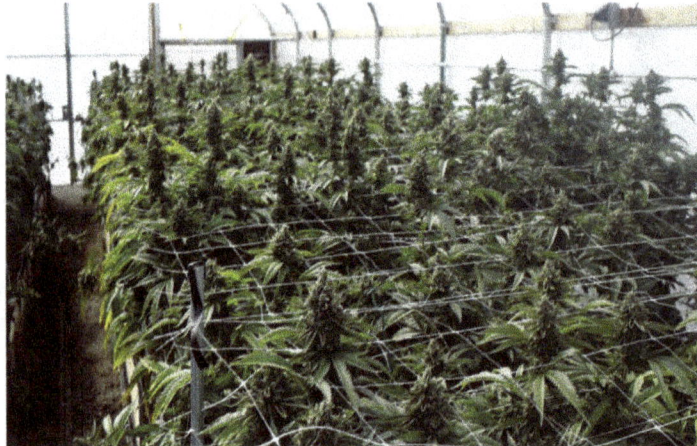

Greenhouse keeps out many bugs

But insects aren't the only pests that can cause problems. This is particularly true if you live in an area that has a large quantity of omnivorous or herbivorous mammals or birds. Deer, rats, rabbits, cows, and other mammals are prone to finding ways to get to your marijuana plants. When the plants are young, it's common for deer to come by and virtually decimate the crop. As the plants age, however, animals aren't as attracted to them.

For large mammals, the best repellent is an equally large fence, but many growers don't have the luxury of being able to build a fence. Thus, other methods are required to force those mammals away. Many growers have started purchasing the urine of certain predators. For instance, if a group of deer constantly messes with your garden, you might think about purchasing some bear urine and placing a perimeter of the stuff around the plants. When the deer catch the scent, they will inherently want to avoid the area from here on out because they recognize the smell as something predatory. This can work for smaller mammals as well. As long as you purchase the urine of one of the mammal's main predators, they will stay away. A rabbit might be repelled by the scent of fox or wolf urine. You can find these repellents at many outdoor shops.

In general, birds don't represent much of a threat to any marijuana garden. When you have just planted the seeds, however, crows, sparrows, and starlings can be potentially harmful to your crop because they like to steal the seeds. This could be a risk until the plant germinates and becomes a seedling. To avoid any of your seeds being taken prematurely, you could use plastic netting or even a scarecrow to keep the birds away.

After the seeds have germinated, you really won't have any problems with birds. They don't really like the taste of the leafy marijuana plant. As mentioned previously, birds should be encouraged to nest in your garden because they are the natural predators of other insect pests.

SOME NOTES ABOUT OUTDOOR SECURITY

Obviously, the difference between growing outdoors and indoors is that outdoors your plants are basically wide open to any onlookers who happen to pass by. If you're on public land (or even private land), there's always a chance that your plants could be found by either law enforcement or thieves. The only way to really prevent yourself from getting caught is to cover your tracks meticulously.

If you're growing on public land, be sure to find a place that will be difficult to discover by land or air. Try to find an area where you know that fly-bys are rare or non-existent. Also, don't plant your garden in an area that is visible from any trails or walking paths.

A random citizen could report your crop to the police and, even if you don't get arrested, you'd likely lose your garden. It's always a good idea to be as clandestine as possible and remain out of the sight of any onlookers (for instance, a park ranger) when you go to the garden. If you can find a place that is secluded but not too hard to reach then you will be much better off when taking care of your plants and ultimately harvesting them.

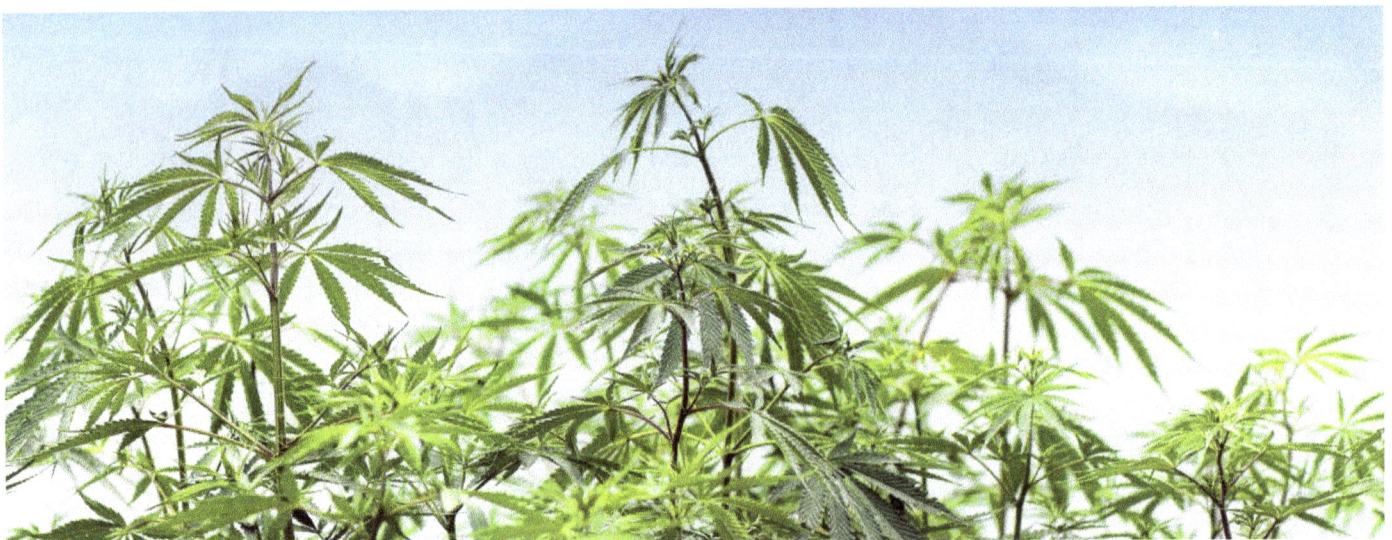

If you have to make a relatively long hike to a place like a clearing in the forest, then it's important to take 3 or 4 different routes. Even an amateur tracker will start to notice the path you make when walking to your garden if you only have one entry point. This path will be obvious to any thieves or other people who know what they're looking for. You should always try to leave your garden in a different way than you came in. For instance, if you are planting in a park with a number of different trails, it could be prudent to enter the park on one trail, leave that trail to tend to your garden, and then leave the garden to get on another trail altogether. Always keep a map of the land handy in the event that you get lost. If it's possible, try entering the public land from inconspicuous places (for instance, areas that don't have trails).

If growing on private land, make sure you do everything in your power to keep the plants from being seen. This includes pruning and trimming them so that they don't invite any suspicion from passersby or neighbors. Plants grown outdoors can often reach incredible heights that will make them relatively obvious to anyone looking. For instance, if you're growing in your backyard, a six-foot monster plant is going to catch the eye of any neighbor relatively quickly. Keeping the plant pruned will limit its size and detectability and might also produce a higher yield in the end.

Some growers have considered growing their crop on land adjacent to their own that is owned by someone else. For example, if you live next to a cornfield, you might think it would be advantageous to grow out there. Unfortunately, it's hard to predict how frequently the landowner inspects their land or if any flybys are performed in the area. If you get caught, expect to be hit with more than a trespassing charge.

It should also be reiterated that you should never talk to anyone about growing marijuana. Even if your plants are heavily secluded and almost impossible to find, don't tell anyone.

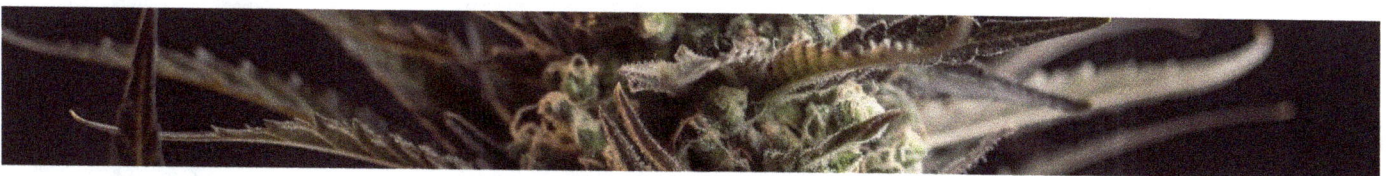

HARVESTING

Indoor and outdoor harvesting are basically the same thing except you have to bring your harvest inside if growing outdoors. If the plants are on private land where you can just pull them out of the ground and bring them in your house then you shouldn't have any trouble. Guerrilla farmers, however, will probably have to hike in to retrieve their plants and then hike back out unnoticed. Of course, this is generally not that easy to do and may require the help of a friend, depending on the size of the plants and the overall size of the crop. If at all possible, try doing this during the night or in the early morning to avoid any chance of people seeing you. Even if you conceal the plants in bags, any onlookers will reach some obvious conclusions.

In any event, taking a few leaves and shoots before the actual harvest time is one of the more prudent decisions you can make. This essentially ensures that you'll at least get something for all your efforts if your plants get stolen or noticed by law enforcement. For indoor growers, it's always good to sample a little bit of the smoke beforehand. The leaves and shoots during vegetative growth will actually be rather potent and will already provide you with a good smoke.

The right time to harvest the plants won't always be apparent. You don't want to harvest too early, and you certainly don't want to harvest too late. In either case, the THC and other cannabinoids on the plant won't be nearly as concentrated as you might like. Obviously, if you want sinsemilla buds, the male plants must be harvested early so they don't pollinate the female flowers. If you remove male flowers early, you won't really be losing that much in terms of potency or yield. For the most part, male plants don't produce the highest quality smoke anyway. Still, if you want to avoid pollination, you should get them out as soon as you determine the sex.

Ready for harvest

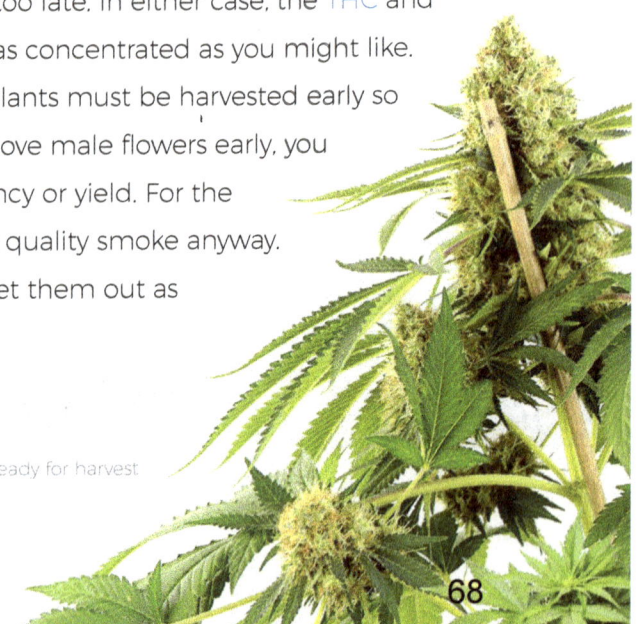

68

If you do want to pollinate your female seeds, then you should just leave the males in the soil so that they can flower and produce pollen. This will keep you from having to pluck out the males prematurely, and it will also ensure that you will have seeds for next year's crop. When it comes to pollinated female plants, you won't want to pull them before the seeds have had enough time to mature. Many growers start to notice the telltale signs of high THC production and increased flower and bud growth, and they might think it's a good idea to pull out their female plants. But, if you pull the plants out too early, the seeds might just be inactive and won't germinate next season. You can investigate the seeds by opening up their sheaths or bracts and seeing if they have achieved the marbling brown color associated with maturity.

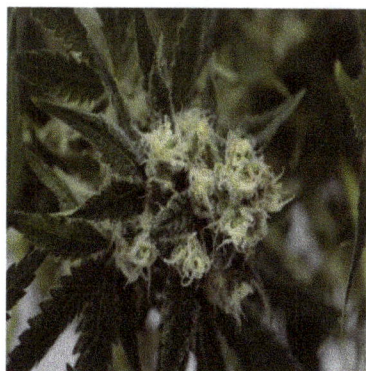

Not ready, white pistils   Ready, many red pistils

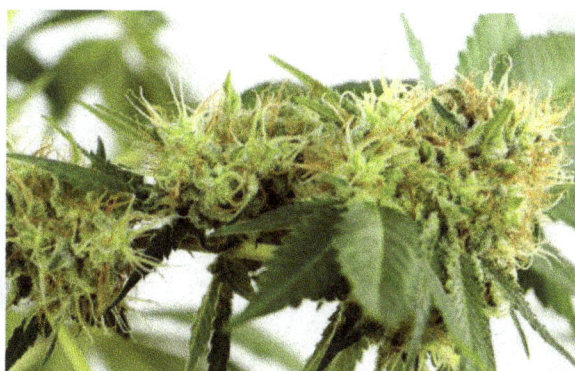

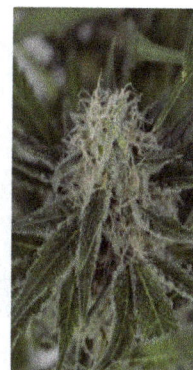

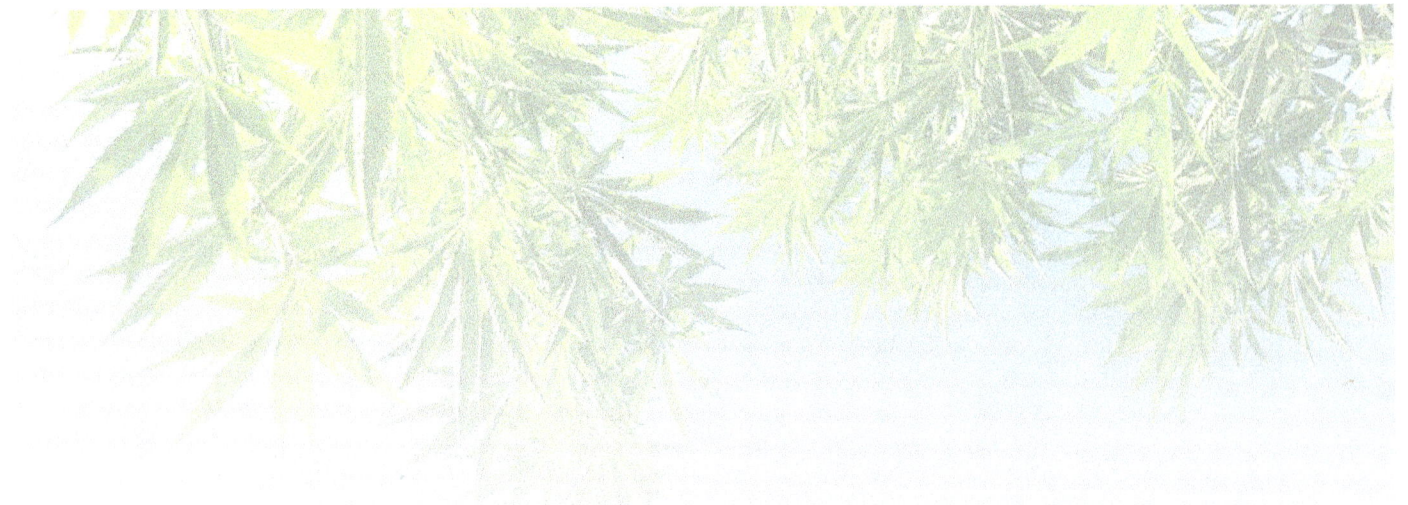

Of course, sinsemilla plants don't have to rely on seed maturation for them to be viable for harvesting. But in general, these plants have a longer flowering period. In fact, they might bloom for 4 to 5 weeks with new growth happening almost instantaneously. The new growth will be sort of a boon to your overall yield, but you should wait until there is a noticeable decline in flower production. This will generally happen in the fourth or fifth week of blooming. When you notice the decline, don't start to harvest immediately. Wait about a week after the decline starts before you start harvesting sinsemilla plants. This is when the THC will be at its highest, and the smoke will be the most potent. If you allow the plants to grow more after this point, they might slowly get a bit larger and produce a few extra buds, but the THC won't be as potent because it will have started to degrade.

To harvest the plants, all you'll have to do is gently pull them up out of the soil. To facilitate this process, you might want to wet the soil beforehand. Avoid bending or cracking the plants as you pull them up, as it makes them harder to deal with. If your plants are in pots you can simply pull them out or even dump the pot and all the soil out.

There are many different techniques of harvesting and transporting marijuana, and I'm always interested in your story.

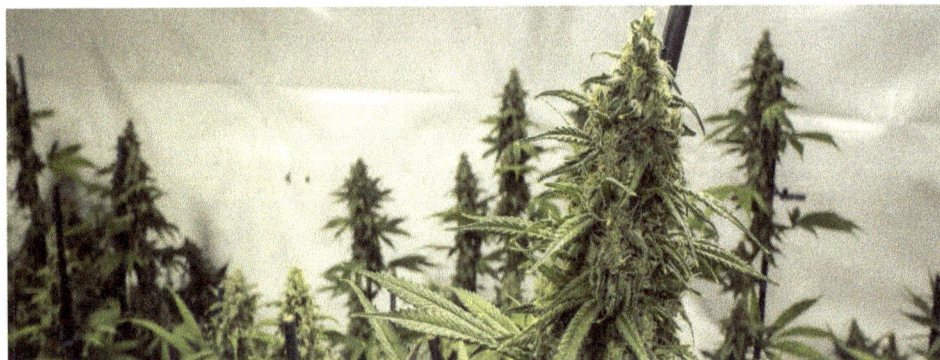

POST-HARVEST ACTIVITIES

When you finally harvest, the first thing you should do is strip the fan leaves off of the plant. This is because they are less potent than the colas and they often don't cure as well as the other parts of the plant. That doesn't mean that they can't be used, however. In fact, fan leaves are known to have a somewhat high concentration of THC, especially after they have just been pulled.

Once you've done that, you can start grading and manicuring the plants. Grading simply involves separating the plants by their particular sex, strain, and anatomical part. For instance, you might place all sativa-dominant, female, top colas in the same area. Most growers like to hang their plants upside down from a wire, if only because it's considerably easier than doing anything else. Manicuring involves taking any excess leaves from around the colas so that the plants will dry quite easily.

After all the plants are graded and manicured neatly, you can start curing them. Curing is a process that is meant to bring out the best flavors and tones, but sometimes it can actually decrease the amount of THC substantially if you do it wrong. Sinsemilla buds often don't require curing because they are potent enough as is.

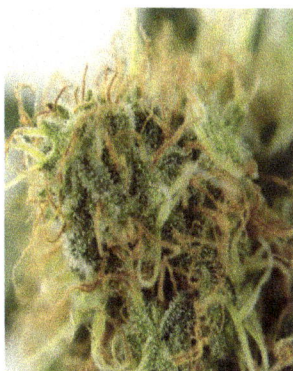
Ready for harvest

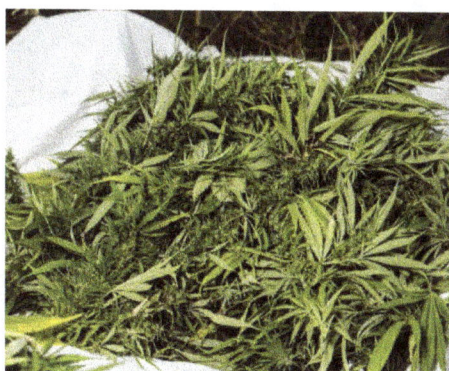
Harvesting

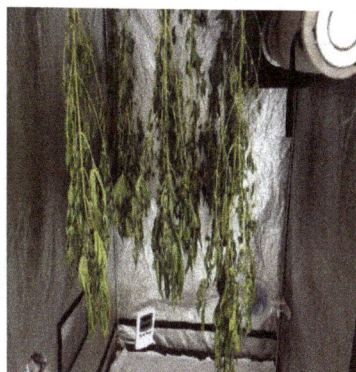
Hang upside down

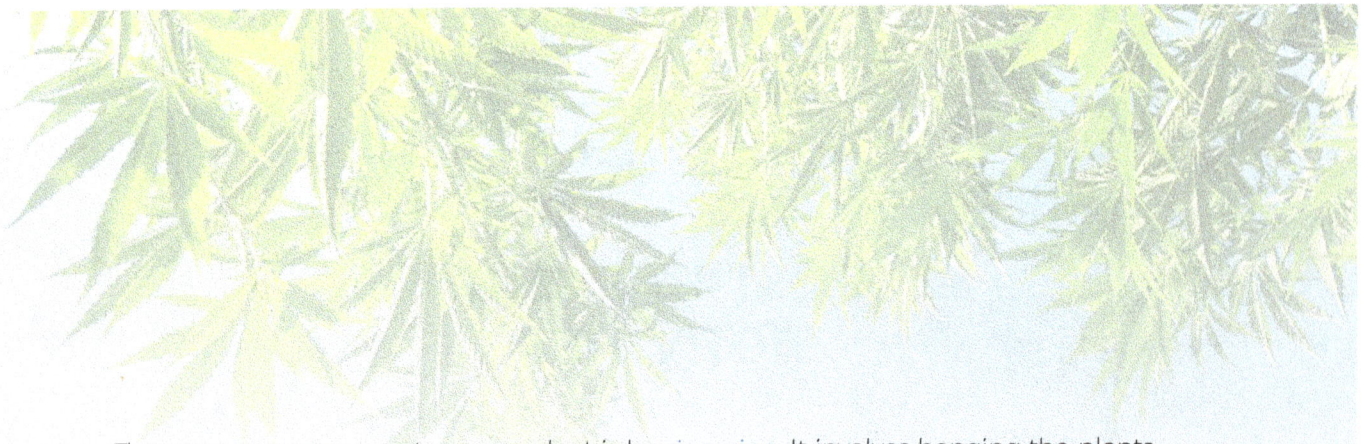

The most common way to cure a plant is by air curing. It involves hanging the plants upside in an unventilated room. You want the temperatures to be relatively hot, so, if you can place the plants in the sun, the curing process should go off without a hitch. The plants will start to lose color and become pale, at which point you should open the ventilator or window to slow down the curing process. The entire length of curing might take you around six weeks to complete. If you are having relatively overcast or wet days or the room isn't staying near 90°F, then you could be at risk of your plants developing mold. This is something you desperately don't want to have happen. To prevent this, you might want to introduce a heater of some kind to keep the temperature as high as it can go.

Flue curing expedites the process of curing by adding an external force that works to heat the plants faster. You can place the plants in a water-tight box that you then place into a pool of water (generally, a fish tank). Then, heat that pool of water to about 90°F consistently. When the plants start to lose their green color, turn the heat up to about 100°F. When all the green is sapped out of the plants, turn the heat up to 115°F. This process will also dry the plants, but make sure to turn the heat down as they start to dry; otherwise, they might end up being brittle. This process generally only takes about a week to complete.

Sweat curing is a method used primarily in Colombia to get the plants to cure within about 5 days. It generally involves stacking branches and colas about 1.5 feet high and 2 square feet minimum. The microbial action works like a fermentation process in the same way that compost starts to heat up. The plants will start to lose color little by little. You should remove the plants that have lost the most color each day. To avoid any mold or rot, place paper towels, cotton sheets, or rags in between each of the plants. The rags will absorb any excess moisture and facilitate the curing process.

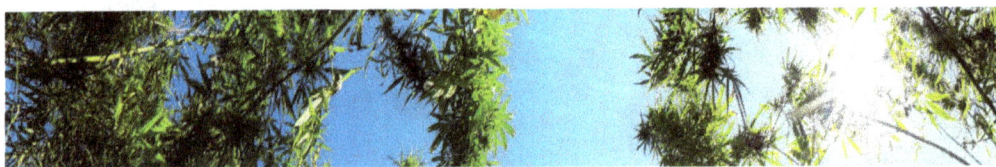

DRYING

At this point, you should start drying your plants. Drying is a necessary activity, particularly if you want to store your bud for later use. It eliminates the risk of incurring mold and also ensures that it lasts a long time. Most growers use a slow drying method that simply involves hanging the plants upside down and letting them air dry naturally.

This usually takes about two weeks to complete. Of course, they will also start to cure a little bit during this process which may limit the potency somewhat.

Fast drying techniques include using the oven, microwaving, and even using a skillet. Most people will want to test out their smoke relatively quickly, and, even though these methods might produce a harsher taste overall, they will still give you the ability to smoke some bud soon after harvesting. It should be noted that you don't want to dry your entire harvest using one of these fast-drying methods. In fact, it might be more prudent to dry the plants using a heater to facilitate the slower drying process. In any event, it's important not to leave marijuana in the oven or skillet for too long. Keep it in the oven for about 10 minutes at a temperature of 150 to 200°F. Don't be careless or you could end up charring your bud entirely.

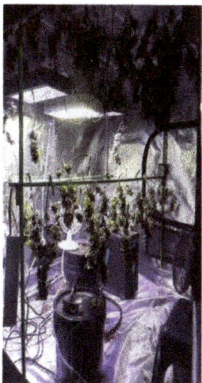

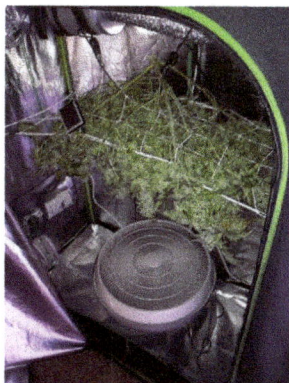

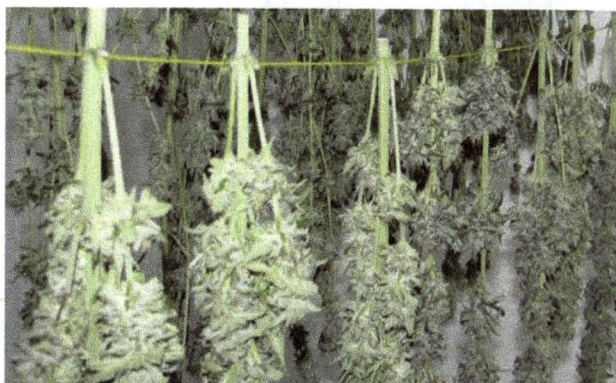

STORAGE

Storing your bud is the best way to ensure that it lasts you until at least the next harvest. Many growers simply place their dried bud in a dark (usually glass) container and then put that container in the refrigerator or freezer. Light and heat are two of the major things that will degrade THC, so if you keep the storage area dark and cold, you will still be able to enjoy your smoke well into the future.

It should also be noted that storing your entire crop in one space is a recipe for disaster. Although it might be more convenient to do it that way, you still run the risk of incurring mold. If even just one portion of one plant stayed moist, you could end up ruining the entire crop with mold. That's why it's important to portion your harvest so that you don't run into a disaster like that.

After that, you can always get ready for next year's crop by tilling some soil or inspecting your seeds. Of course, you could also just sit back, relax, and enjoy the fruits of your labor for a while. Hopefully, this Grow Bible helped you through the process of growing your marijuana crop, and it will continue to support you as you keep growing for years to come.

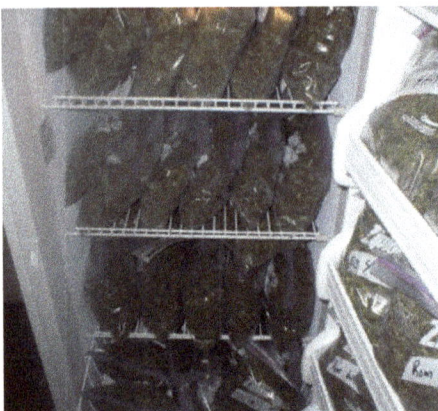

Airtight jars

MARIJUANA PLANT CARE

NUTRIENT PROBLEMS FOR MARIJUANA PLANTS

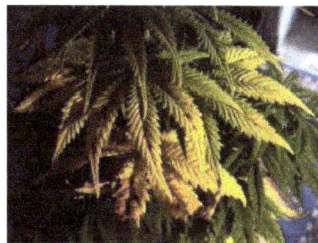

With marijuana, nutrient issues can crop constantly. The three major nutrients that you'll be dealing with are nitrogen, phosphorus, and potassium (or, N, P, and K). Of course, other micronutrients like magnesium, zinc, or calcium can also play a role in nutrient problems or deficiencies. The biggest issue that marijuana growers will have to contend with is maintaining an accurate pH balance in the water and soil. The pH number is largely responsible for how many nutrients the marijuana plants absorb.

Adjusting the pH balance is generally a matter of making it more acidic or more alkaline. You want the pH to be near the middle of the pH scale between 6.0 and 7.0. Every nutrient that you add or subtract from the soil can affect the pH balance and what the plant will be able to use in terms of nutrients. Understanding that can help you keep healthy marijuana plants for a long time.

PH LEVELS FOR MARIJUANA PLANTS

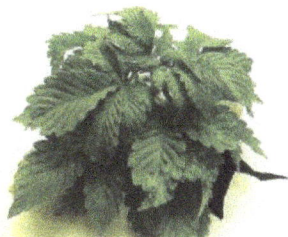

The pH scale is a measure of how acidic or alkaline a substance is. It ranges from 1.0 to 14.0 where 7.0 is neutral. The lower on the scale a substance is, the higher its acidity. The higher on the scale, the higher its alkalinity. In terms of watering marijuana, you want to make sure that both the water and the soil you're using are at an appropriate level. In soil, the ideal pH number is between 6.0 and 6.5, and in hydroponic systems, marijuana will grow with a low pH of 5.5, but the 6.0 to 6.5 range is still the best for marijuana plants to absorb nutrients.

Testing the pH level is as simple as purchasing test strips. It's important to keep the pH at an acceptable level to avoid the risk of nutrient deficiency. To avoid pH problems with soil, you can purchase commercial mixes that are created to stay at ideal pH levels. Otherwise,

MARIJUANA PLANT CARE

using items like pH-Up and pH-Down will get you into the desirable range.

MARIJUANA NUTRIENT DEFICIENCY – BORON

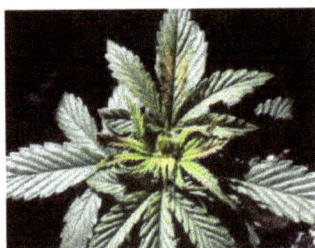

Boron deficiency is rare when you're growing marijuana, but it can affect the plant's ability to thrive. The first sign of a boron deficiency comes with the growing tips turning brown or gray. In fact, the only thing that a boron deficiency really affects in the marijuana plant is new growth. The growing tips will eventually start to die, but you'll also see dead spots scattered across the leaves. The dead spots aren't very large, however.

In any event, you really want to treat the problem, because boron is important for plant processes like seed formation, pollen production, and other plant-building functions. Fixing the problem is generally a matter of using certain irrigation practices. Using boric acid is the easiest step, but you can also make use of compost, compost teas, or borax to get the boron levels back to normal.

MARIJUANA NUTRIENT DEFICIENCY – CALCIUM

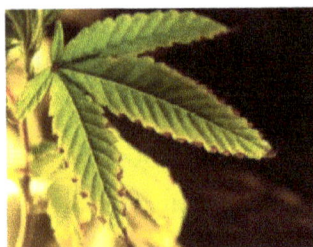

Calcium deficiency is uncommon in marijuana plants that are grown outside, but it can occur when the plant is grown in planting mixes and, most commonly, in hydroponics. Certain types of water are not composed of large amounts of calcium making them unfit for using in hydroponic systems. If you're only using water and a nutrient solution, then you might not be getting enough calcium to the marijuana plants. Calcium deficiencies generally manifest as big, necrotic blotches on leaves that have turned dark green.

MARIJUANA PLANT CARE

Older growth is affected the most, and the branches are weakened to the point that they may be easy to crack. A calcium deficiency can also end up affecting the root system if it's not handled early on. Treating a calcium deficiency requires the use of a calcium-rich substance like lime. Infusing that into the plant system can help it regain strength in the older growth and in the roots.

MARIJUANA NUTRIENT DEFICIENCY – COPPER

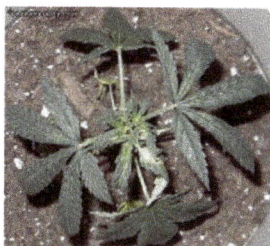

Although copper deficiencies are uncommon, they can hurt new growth quite substantially. A deficiency in this type of element will produce necrosis in young leaves. This will also cause the leaves to turn a copper-like or bluish gray color at the tips. New growth can also be affected when flowers start to appear. So, you may get limp leaves, flowers, and other plant parts if copper is in short supply.

Because copper is so important for reproduction and maturity, you're going to want to give the plant something that will replenish the copper.

MARIJUANA NUTRIENT DEFICIENCY – IRON

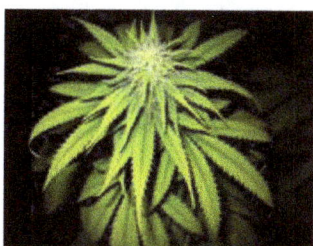

It's somewhat common for marijuana plants to experience an iron deficiency. It will affect new growth in the plant, including leaves. For the most part, upper leaves will be affected, and you'll start to notice a distinct yellowing in those leaves. The veins will stay green, but the leaves themselves will not have the right amount of chlorophyll. In fact, iron plays a large part in the creation of chlorophyll in the marijuana plant.

An iron deficiency can look a lot like a magnesium deficiency, except that iron only effects new growth. So, the issues will take place only in the top leaves and not the lower- to mid-range leaves. Iron deficiencies generally occur in tandem with an imbalanced pH level, so you need to adjust for that when you treat the deficiency. It can also occur simultaneously with zinc and manganese deficiencies. Learn more about iron deficiencies and how to treat them.

MARIJUANA NUTRIENT DEFICIENCY – MAGNESIUM

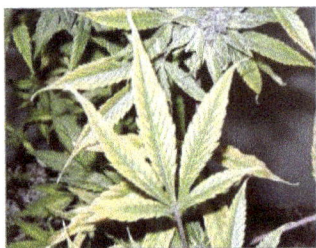

A magnesium deficiency is rare when you're growing marijuana outside, but it can happen in indoor soil and soilless mediums. It primarily affects the lower leaves of the plant at first, turning them yellow and making them lose vigor. Eventually, these leaves will die. The deficiency will work its way up to the middle and then the top layer of leaves. The element is a major factor in the production of chlorophyll in the plant and it's important to infuse your marijuana plant with magnesium if it exhibits these symptoms.

Epsom salts are the quickest and easiest way to treat a magnesium deficiency. It's also important to distinguish between a magnesium deficiency and iron deficiency so that you don't end up over-fertilizing the plants.

Marijuana Plant Care

MARIJUANA NUTRIENT DEFICIENCY – MANGANESE

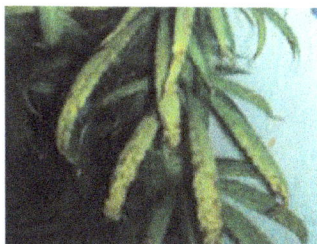

Manganese deficiencies are rather uncommon in marijuana plants. They are almost always found in conjunction with iron and zinc deficiencies, so you have to keep that in mind when treating the plants. The deficiency will appear in new leaves. These leaves will start to turn yellow and exhibit several necrotic spots. The vigor in the plant can be severely decreased when manganese is not present in high enough quantities. On the flip side, too much manganese can actually cause an iron deficiency.

Manganese is important for chlorophyll production and creating nitrates. Thus, it's important to ensure that you have proper levels of manganese in the soil or nutrient solution that you are providing the plants. Water-soluble fertilizer works well as a way to infuse the soil with manganese. Greensand and compost are also good options.

MARIJUANA NUTRIENT DEFICIENCY – MOLYBDENUM

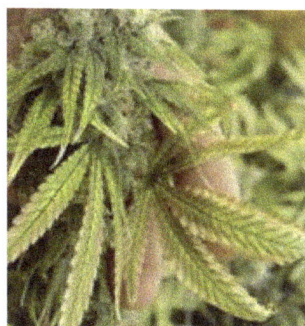

Deficiencies in molybdenum are not common at all, but they can produce some strange effects in the marijuana plant. If you don't have enough molybdenum, you will start to notice that the middle leaves will yellow. Any new growth will also start to turn up warped or it will be stopped altogether. The shoots will start twisting and the leaves may exhibit a sort of red discoloration at the tips. Molybdenum's job is to aid in the production of ammonia which is vital for other plant functions.

The reason why molybdenum deficiencies are rare in marijuana plants is because the plants don't need a lot of the element. So, to treat any deficiency you can use a foliar spray or just

Marijuana Plant Care

add molybdenum-infused solutions to the hydroponic system. If you want more information on <u>molybdenum deficiencies in marijuana</u>, just click through.

MARIJUANA NUTRIENT DEFICIENCY – NITROGEN

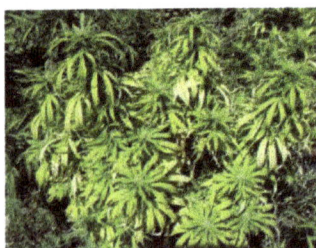

Because nitrogen is one of the most common nutrients that you'll find in marijuana, it's also common for it to be deficient in some way. Nitrogen plays an important role in many of the plant's functions including the production of amino acids and the vitality of photosynthesis. Any deficiencies of nitrogen in the marijuana plant will manifest themselves first in the yellowing of the leaves. The leaves will start to curl in and die if the deficiency isn't treated fast. The deficiency works its way up from the bottom leaves to the top leaves.

Correcting a nitrogen deficiency is all about using the right fertilizer with the right NPK ratio. Obviously, you want the "N" number to be higher during most of the vegetative growth.

MARIJUANA NUTRIENT DEFICIENCY – PHOSPHORUS

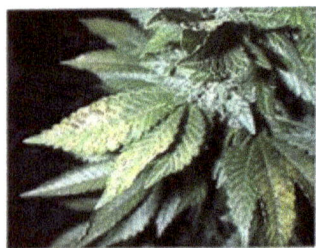

Growing marijuana rarely yields plants that are deficient in phosphorus, but it is a possibility. The plant will start to exhibit symptoms like darkening leaf colors and slow growth. Over time, the leaves will start to curve back toward the plant and turn a tannish, brown color. Petioles and other plant parts start exhibiting darker, blue or red colors. Phosphorus is most important during the flowering period as a reproductive agent, but it also helps strengthen

MARIJUANA PLANT CARE

the root system and the stems. If there is not enough phosphorus during the flowering period, the marijuana plants may not yield at their highest capacity.

To eliminate the phosphorus deficiency, you need to find a fertilizer that has an NPK ratio with a higher amount of P. Bloom fertilizers and high-phosphorus guano can effectively mitigate the effect of the phosphorus deficiency. Use a water-soluble variety for the best results.

MARIJUANA NUTRIENT DEFICIENCY – POTASSIUM

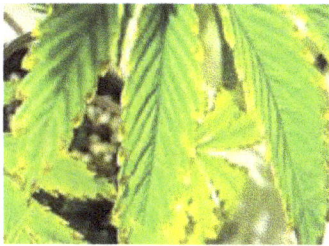

Potassium deficiencies in marijuana are somewhat common. When using natural fertilizers like guano, you have to take into account the fact that potassium is going to be the least abundant of the three macronutrients (nitrogen and phosphorus being the other two). A potassium deficiency might actually make the marijuana plants appear taller and more vigorous at first glance, but the bottom leaves might be dying. The leaves may also be turning a tan or brown color and developing necrotic spots in some locations.

Chlorotic spots will start to show up as the deficiency persists. Slow growth and smaller growth are all possibilities with a potassium deficiency. Potassium is important in the transport of water and the development of buds later on. Even so, small deficiencies are really only cosmetic.

MARIJUANA PLANT CARE

MARIJUANA NUTRIENT DEFICIENCY – SILICON

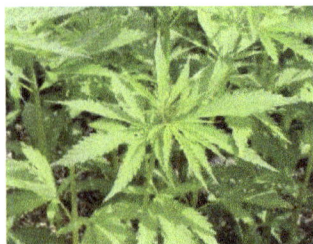

Silicon deficiencies in marijuana are quite rare, largely because silicon is generally an abundant element in nature. It's also relatively abundant in any nutrient solutions, fertilizers, or other plant helpers that you might have. Because silicon plays a large role in plant production, a silicon deficiency will produce less sturdy stems and branches. Silicon is also a natural insect deterrent. You may notice that insects are more attracted to your marijuana plant. Photosynthesis is also affected negatively with a silicon shortage.

There are a few sources of silicon that will fix a silicon deficiency. These include diatomaceous earth and even liquid silicon. Again, however, silicon deficiencies are rare and you may be better off looking at other sources for your plant's problems.

MARIJUANA NUTRIENT DEFICIENCY – SULFUR

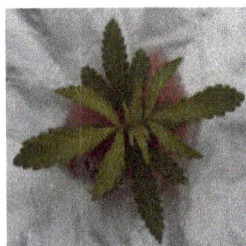

Although sulfur deficiencies are rare, they do still occasionally happen. The marijuana plant will start to exhibit signs of sulfur deficiency with the yellowing of newer leaves. The growth can become stunted and the leaves narrower and more brittle than before. It's important to keep sulfur at an acceptable level because it assists in a number of different plant processes including root growth and chlorophyll production.

The reason that sulfur shortages rarely occur, though, is that most fertilizers and soils have a naturally acceptable amount of sulfur in them. That means you'll rarely encounter plants that have a sulfur deficiency. If you do get sulfur deficient marijuana plants, then correcting the problem is rather easy. Epsom salts, potassium sulfate, and several other remedies can get the job done if you're experiencing any of the symptoms related to sulfur deficiency.

MARIJUANA PLANT CARE

MARIJUANA NUTRIENT DEFICIENCY – ZINC

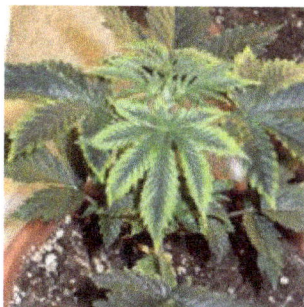

Zinc deficiencies in marijuana are somewhat common and they produce some noticeable changes in the structure of the plant. The leaf blades on the new growth will be twisted and the older leaves' veins will start to turn yellow. The plant will also turn slightly pale on some occasions. During flowering, buds will start to twist and be misshapen. Zinc deficiency is generally linked to deficiencies in both manganese and iron.

Zinc is helpful in a number of ways including plant-building and enzyme production. A severe lack of zinc can cause the plant to wilt or be brittle. To fix a zinc deficiency, you need to keep both manganese and iron in mind. Because these three are often linked, the best course of action is to get a micro mix of all three. That way you can cover all your bases.

PESTS

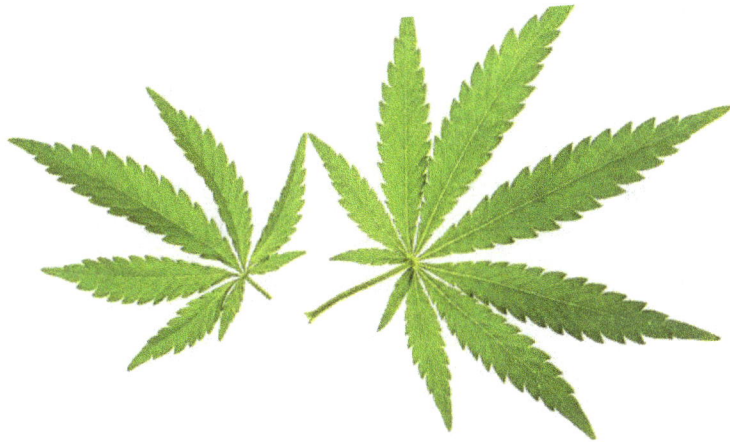

Marijuana Plant Care

PESTS AND BUGS PROBLEM SOLVER FOR MARIJUANA PLANTS

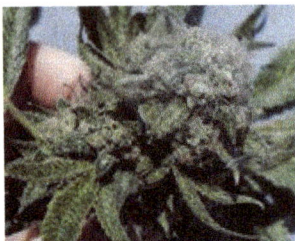

Pests and bugs are major problems for a variety of cannabis plants. All sorts of little critters enjoy the taste of marijuana plants and they could end up ruining an entire crop if an infestation appears. Ants, caterpillars, mealybugs, and spider mites are all pests that can have an effect on your marijuana crop. Using chemical pesticides might seem like an easy option, but it can actually be harmful in the long run. The chemicals are likely unsafe for inhalation or ingestion by humans, even if they get rid of the bug problem.

Thus, it's important to use organic deterrents like introducing pest predators into the environment or using a natural remedy. In some cases, the best pesticide is preemptive defense. Although indoor marijuana gardens are technically less susceptible to pets, you can inadvertently introduce a population of plant killers by bringing them in on your clothes. So, it's always good to be careful when dealing with pests and bugs. Click here for the entire pest and bug section.

MARIJUANA PESTS – ANTS

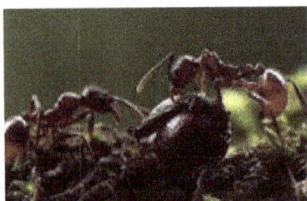

Ants don't technically pose a threat to your cannabis garden, but they are an indicator of an underlying threat that you may not notice. Ants are attracted to marijuana not because they like the taste of the plant, but because the aphids and whiteflies that populate the plant produce a sweet nectar that the ants like to munch on. So, when you see ants in and around your cannabis garden, they might not be doing much damage themselves, but they are protecting the pests that actually do a lot of damage.

Even so, the ants and their soil mounds can affect the root system of the plants and you'll want to eradicate them. You can do this in a number of ways, but cornmeal seems to be

MARIJUANA PLANT CARE

the most effect ant killer that you'll find.

MARIJUANA PESTS – APHIDS

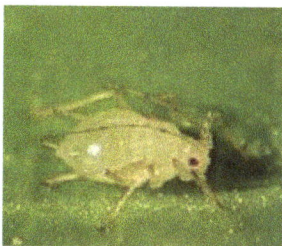

Aphids are one of the peskiest bug problems you can incur and they are sometimes hard to notice. These little pale, yellow creatures hang around on the underside of the leaves, sucking them dry of their nutrients and reproducing at a rate of 12 offspring per day. If you're growing marijuana indoors, aphids can almost entirely wipe out your garden if they go unchecked. Outdoors, however, Mother Nature tends to balance out the ratio. Parasitic wasps and ladybugs are predators of aphids but in different ways.

A good indicator that you might have aphids is the presence of ants. Ants are not attracted to marijuana on its own, but the aphids produce a nectar that the ants like. If you want to get rid of an aphid infestation, then there are a number of different organic remedies at your disposal. Most of these come in the form of sprays that you can make in your own home.

MARIJUANA PESTS – BIRDS

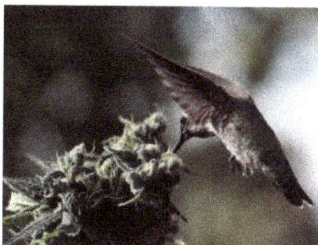

Under most circumstances, birds will actually help keep pests out of your outdoor marijuana garden. They like to eat caterpillars, worms, and other creatures that might enjoy your marijuana leaves. But, birds can also seek to end your marijuana garden before it's really even started. Many birds enjoy marijuana seeds, and, if you're not careful, you could have a flock of birds

Marijuana Plant Care

poaching your pre-germinated collection. The last thing you want is to lose your marijuana seeds before they've even produced a single sprout.

To <u>stop the birds</u> from eliminating your garden, there are a few things that you can try. Scarecrows, shiny objects, or netting over the marijuana seeds all help deter birds from getting to your seeds. Just remember that you'll want those birds around when the plants start to thrive. They only produce benefits when the plants are nice and green and attractive to a wide variety of different bugs.

MARIJUANA PESTS – CATERPILLARS

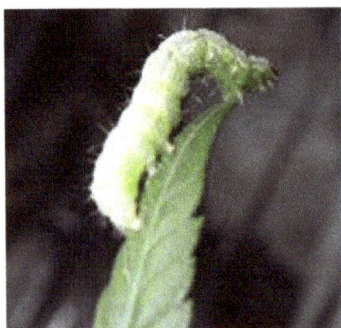

Caterpillars are some of the most dangerous pests to your crops. They are both voracious eaters and hard to notice sometimes. This is especially true in the case of corn borers or hemp borers. These little creatures eat the stems and stalks from the inside out. You may not even be aware that they're doing it because they literally bore a hole into the location and stay out of sight. It's feasible for borers to hollow out an entire marijuana plant until it falls over on itself.

Other caterpillars that are content to stay on the outside of the plant can still ruin sections if you're not careful. Virtually all caterpillars enjoy the taste of marijuana. The prevalence of caterpillars is curbed by praying mantises and parasitic wasps, but you can also use organic remedies to get the caterpillars to move on.

MARIJUANA PLANT CARE

MARIJUANA PESTS – CATS AND DOGS

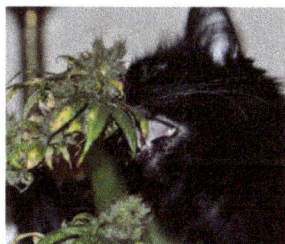

Although you may love your pets, they still might mess up some of your cannabis crop, but maybe not in the way that you think. Cats and dogs aren't usually attracted to marijuana as a food source, but they are known for doing their business wherever they might please. Urine and fecal excrement are both things that you want to keep away from your still-growing marijuana garden. This also might sound counterintuitive considering that both urine and fecal matter can be fertilizers, but they both cause more problems than you might be aware of.

Cat urine is known to be high in ammonia which has a negative effect on marijuana plants. Additionally, fecal matter from your dog or cat can attract the wrong kind of parasites to your marijuana garden. Beyond that, cats and dogs like to mess things up, so be sure to keep them away from the garden or make them understand that it is not an area for playing around.

MARIJUANA PESTS – CUTWORMS

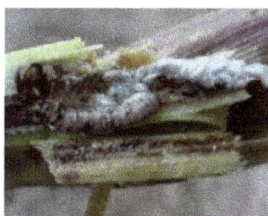

Cutworms are most dangerous to your marijuana garden when it's at a young age. Seedlings can be entirely wiped out cutworms if you're not careful. The worst part about cutworms is that they really only work under the cover of darkness, so you may never notice them until it's too late. If the tops of the seedlings look like they've been cut and you haven't actually been cutting them, then there's a good chance that you have cutworms.

Getting rid of cutworms isn't that hard, though. The bugs are naturally susceptible to several predators and they can be wiped out without any human intervention. Other methods of removing a cutworm population include tilling the soil or planting sunflowers on the perimeter of your marijuana garden. Tilling allows you to root out the population while sunflowers will keep the critters at bay until the marijuana plants are big enough to not be threatened by cutworms.

MARIJUANA PESTS – CRICKETS AND GRASSHOPPERS

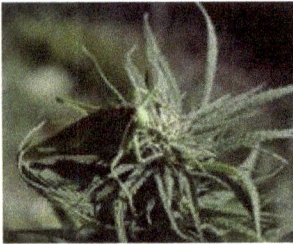

Crickets and grasshoppers can cause major problems for your marijuana crop. They are omnivorous little creatures that will eat just about anything you put in front of them. If left unchecked, a marijuana plant can become the staple of their diet. There are many different types of crickets (including mole crickets) that can wreak havoc on your garden. They are also mostly nocturnal, meaning that a lot of their meals occur after you've gone to bed.

Fixing a cricket infestation is tough because they can be hard to notice, but you don't often want to rely on natural factors. Because some the bugs live in mounds under the earth, they attract mammals and birds who will gladly dig them up. This can be detrimental to your crop because it can expose the root systems. The best way to get rid of crickets and grasshoppers is to use a mixture of water and dishwashing liquid.

MARIJUANA PESTS – DEER

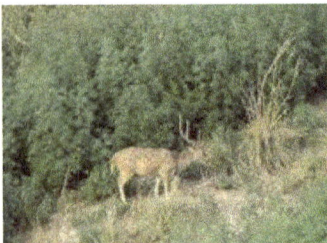

Deer are herbivores who eat just about any kind of greenery that you put in front of them. But, they do have a taste palate and won't come near marijuana plants as they start to mature and gain more cannabinoids. Until that point, however, deer are actually quite fond of the cannabis plant and it's important to keep them away as best you can. Obviously, the best defense is

MARIJUANA PLANT CARE

to actually put up a fence. This acts as a physical barrier between the deer and the plants, and they will most often look for food elsewhere.

If that's not an option, you can always use one of the many other options that will scare off deer. For instance, bright lights are known to startle a curious doe here and there. You can also use scents that will deter the deer. Something like garlic or moth balls will generally keep any deer population at arm's length.

MARIJUANA PESTS – FUNGUS GNATS

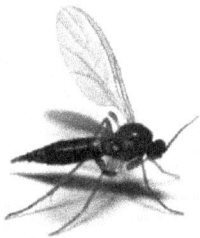

Fungus gnats don't have a particularly friendly-sounding name and there's good reason for that. They could potentially cause major damage to your cannabis crop if you're not careful. Both the adults and their microscopic larvae are known to chow down on marijuana plants. The bugs start feeding on fungus at the base of the plant, but will eventually make their way into the root system. This causes plant growth to slow and vigor to reduce. Fungus gnats also cause major problems with the drainage of the soil.

Checking for fungus gnats is as simple as putting out a sticky pad near the base of the marijuana plant, but that won't totally eradicate the problem. You'll likely still have larvae wriggling around in the soil and a mixture of peroxide mixed in with the water will generally do the trick.

MARIJUANA PLANT CARE

MARIJUANA PESTS – GOPHERS AND MOLES

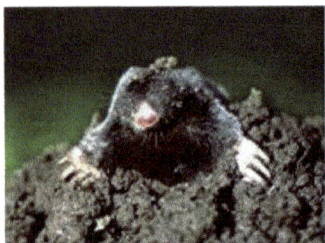

Gophers and moles both spend a lot of their time underground. They burrow underneath and create tunnels and small living spaces for themselves and other critters. Moles generally don't pose much of a threat to cannabis because they are not interested in the plants, at all. Instead, they'll just aerate the soil for you and potentially kill off any bugs in the area. Gophers, though, are much more dangerous to cannabis plants. Instead of working around the root system, they will actually eat the roots. They may even grab entire plants and bring them down into their tunnels for dinner.

So, it's a good idea to try and avoid gophers as best as possible. They have natural predators like owls and hawks, but, if neither of those are around, you can use garlic or castor oil to get the gophers to move to another location. Find out more about gophers and moles here.

MARIJUANA PESTS – LEAF MINERS

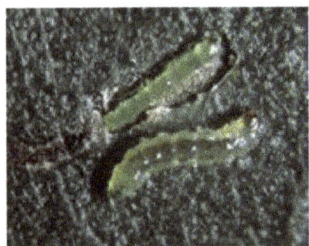

Leaf miners, as you might expect, tend to "mine" the leaves of the marijuana plant for their nutrients. They leave rather obvious white or brown streaks on the tops of the marijuana leaves. As adults, leaf miners look like the common housefly, but they are certainly much more dangerous. They plant their larvae onto the underside of the leaves and then the larvae themselves burrow into the plants.

The only effective way to get rid of these creatures is to actually smash them on your own. Pesticides are ineffective and, of course, you may end up doing more harm than good. Find out more about leaf miners here.

Marijuana Plant Care

MARIJUANA PESTS – MEALY BUGS

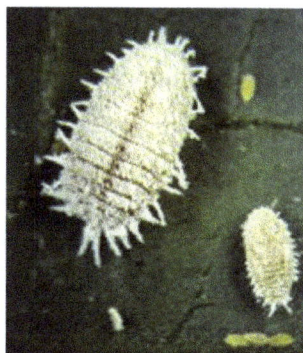

Mealy bugs are small, pale little creatures that hang out around the crevices of the marijuana plant. In small portions, mealy bugs don't cause a lot of harm, but they need to be controlled if their population starts to balloon. One of the biggest signs of a mealy bug infestation is the incidence of white, cotton-like balls of stuff that the bugs deposit. You will also start to notice droopy leaves with blotches on them.

One of the things that keeps mealy bugs around is the protection of ants. If you find ants around your marijuana garden, then there's a good chance that you also have an infestation of mealy bugs. There are a number of ways to get rid of mealy bugs including taking them off physically or using homemade remedies.

MARIJUANA PESTS – RATS AND MICE

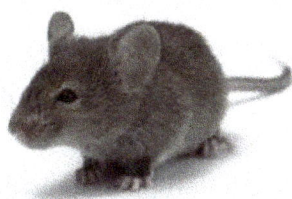

Rats and mice will eat just about anything you put in front of them. Obviously, they're more inclined to actual human food than they are to plant material, but if no food is available, then they might opt for cannabis plants. Even if they're not hungry, they might just use the cannabis stalks and stems as a way to control their constantly growing teeth. Because they are very sneaky and don't like to be seen, it's hard to actually catch a mouse or rat in the act.

The best way to avoid a rat or mouse infestation is to create an environment that is unwelcoming to them. Of course, if you have any hawks or other flesh-eating birds in the neighborhood, then you really won't have to worry. In essence, you just want to deter the rodents from coming around because they don't generally pose much of a threat.

MARIJUANA PLANT CARE

MARIJUANA PESTS – SNAILS AND SLUGS

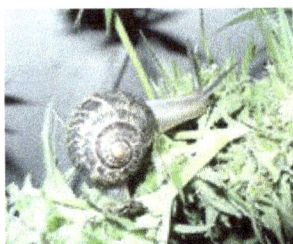

Snails and slugs are a common problem for outdoor marijuana. We're all familiar with the gloopy trail of silver that they leave behind and you'll know when they come along. Both snails and slugs are frequent diners at marijuana gardens and they can severely damage a plant if left to their own devices for too long. Their natural predators are frogs and toads, so creating an environment that is attractive to the amphibians is a good preventative measure.

If that's out of the question or you have already been infested with snails and slugs, then there are many ways to deal with the problem. Obviously, salt is a big killer of snails and slugs, but you can also get rid of them with a number of innovative measures.

MARIJUANA PESTS – SPIDER MITES

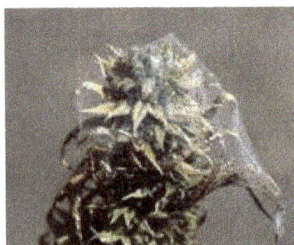

One of the biggest problems that you can face with a marijuana garden is spider mites. Spider mites are very fast reproducers and they reach adulthood in only around five days. So, it's easy to be bombarded with the pests in a short period of time. Spider mites generally feed on the plants, extracting chlorophyll in great quantities until the plant is sapped of all its energy. This can potentially ruin entire crops if it goes unchecked.

There are plenty of natural remedies to this issue, including the introduction of some spider mite predators like ladybugs. If you don't have any ladybugs available, then you can actually buy some to curb the population of spider mites. You may also be able to simply spray the spider mites off the plants with a hose (if that's feasible) or a water and neem oil spray. They will be incapable of moving and will starve to death underneath the marijuana plants.

MARIJUANA PLANT CARE

MARIJUANA PESTS – THRIPS

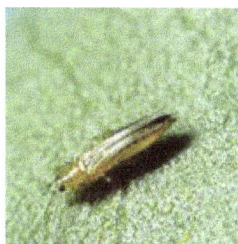

Thrips are very small insects, but they can cause huge problems with your marijuana garden. They feed primarily on incipient flowers, meaning that the maturation process of the plants will be severely curtailed. They are also known to be disease vectors, spreading viruses from one plant to the next. These can be potentially more deadly than the thrips themselves.

Avoiding thrips is all about practice good preventative maintenance. Using a high-quality compost can be a good way to avoid thrip infestation. If the thrips have already invaded your garden then you will obviously need other means by which to eliminate them. They do have several natural predators, like predatory mites, that can curb the infestation. You can also just shake the plants if you notice a thrip infestation or spray them with a mixture of water and neem oil.

MARIJUANA PESTS – WHITEFLIES

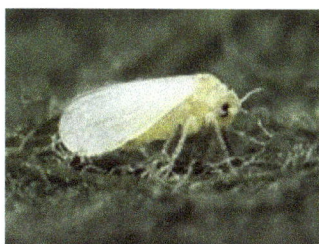

Whiteflies are small, but highly detrimental creatures that can wipe out an entire crop if you're not careful. They hide on the bottom of the leaves munching on the green material and potentially spreading diseases. In fact, that is their major drawback: the propensity to be a vector for disease. The bigger problem is that they are highly mobile so the extent of their disease-carrying abilities is far and wide. The best way to combat whiteflies to make sure they never show up in the first place.

The best way to do this is by encouraging the natural predators of the whitefly to show up in droves. Planting flowers like zinnias is a good way to attract hummingbirds and predatory insects. This is something that should keep the whiteflies away. If it doesn't, you can always try natural concoctions using items like garlic to shoo the whiteflies away.

DISEASES

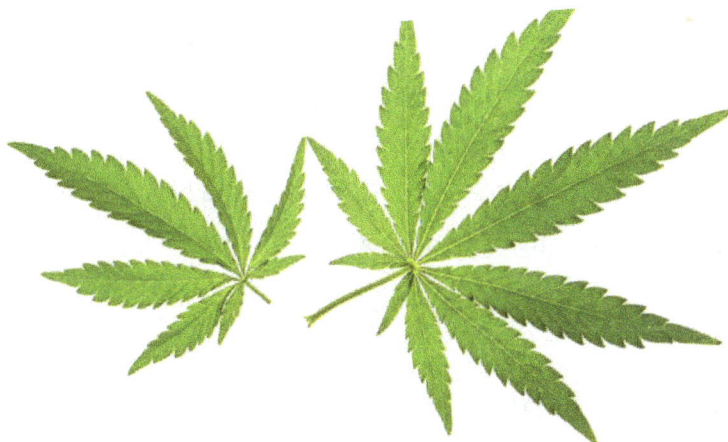

MARIJUANA PLANT CARE

DISEASES AFFECTING CANNABIS – IDENTIFICATION AND CONTROL

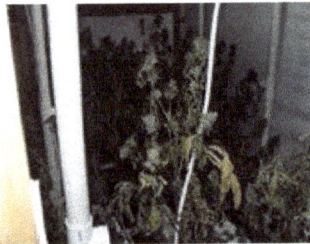

Diseases are some of the worst cannabis problems that you'll encounter. Marijuana diseases come in two categories: fungal and bacterial. Fungal diseases are usually the result of conditions that are too humid or damp. Fungal spores float around in the air looking for an ideal location to spread themselves. Oftentimes, that location can be on your cannabis plant.

Bacterial infections are often subtler in the way they attack. They can be introduced by a number of different vectors including bugs, humans, and even rain. Bacteria won't infect healthy marijuana plants right away, but if they find an opening, they can take down an entire plant. It's important to understand the signs of a fungal or bacterial disease in marijuana so that you can properly treat it when it occurs. As always, the best defense against disease is prevention, so creating a space that is unattractive to fungus and bacteria is vital.

MARIJUANA DISEASES – ALGAE

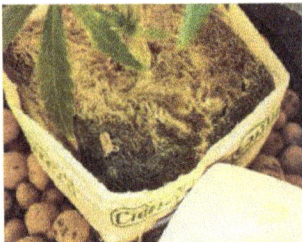

Algae is a common problem in hydroponic systems, largely because both marijuana and algae thrive under those conditions. But, you don't want any algae sharing space with your marijuana plants. Algae tends to attach itself to the roots of the plant which deprives marijuana of the valuable nutrients it needs to thrive in a hydroponic system.

Again, the best defense against algae is taking proper precautions beforehand. Because algae requires light and moisture to grow efficiently, it's hard to make the conditions in a hydroponic system unattractive. The best way to dissuade algae growth in your marijuana grow room is to use dark or opaque material with your growing apparatuses. If you have an infestation of algae, there are a number of things that you can do—including cleaning out

Marijuana Plant Care

the reservoir—to get back on the right track.

MARIJUANA DISEASES – GRAY MOLD, BUD ROT OR BOTRYTIS

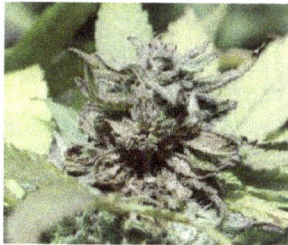

Gray mold is perhaps the single most detrimental issue you can face as a cannabis grower. It infects virtually every part of the plant, from the stems and stalks to the buds and flowers. It does not discriminate between the parts of the plant that it enjoys. It's very important to avoid introducing gray mold into your environment. The disease is most comfortable in cool or temperate environments where humidity is present in some degree. Try to keep the temperature in the grow room above 70*F and keep down the humidity as best as you can.

You can also go above and beyond by changing clothes before you step into the grow room. Spores can sometimes latch onto clothing and then be released in the marijuana grow room when they've found a suitable host. There are several sprays or soaps that you can use if the plant is already infected.

MARIJUANA DISEASES – LEAF SEPTORIA – YELLOW LEAF SPOT

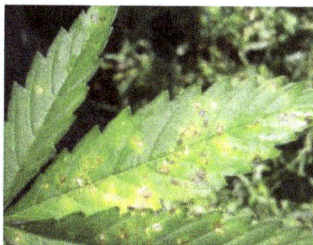

Yellow leaf spot, as you might expect, produces yellow spots on the leaves of your cannabis plants. It is a fungal disease that mostly shows up on outdoor marijuana plants that have been exposed to warmth and rain simultaneously. Spots will start to appear on lower leaves first, before working their way upward. In severe cases, an entire leaf might turn yellow and then start to crumble away. For the most part, only leaves and occasionally stems will be affected and your crop as a whole won't be endangered because of yellow leaf spot.

Still, yellow leaf spot can decrease yield and it's important to avoid it at all costs. Preventing yellow leaf spot is all a matter of using sterile gardening practices. For instance, you should always till the ground thoroughly and maybe even use a fungicide in the compost so that yellow leaf spot is dissuaded. If that doesn't work and you still get yellow leaf spot on your plants, then there is a way to beat it using a mixture of baking soda and other practices.

MARIJUANA DISEASES – POWDERY MILDEW

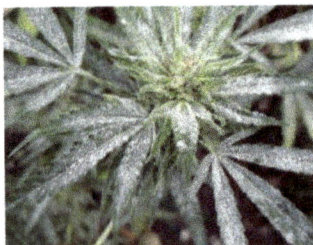

Powdery mildew is something that can keep plaguing your marijuana garden time and time again. It can affect both indoor and outdoor gardens because the spores are carried on the wind. The worst part about powdery mildew is that it is sneakier than you might imagine. The spores can just lie in waiting until conditions are ideal for them to "take up root." Mildew thrives in conditions in which the humidity level is above 55% and the temperatures are generally warm.

Mildew is also common in marijuana plants that are positioned too close to one another. If you have an overcrowded grow room, then you could be risking the lives of your plants. Powdery mildew generally has a white color and affects the leaves and the plant's ability to photosynthesize. If you have incurred a powdery mildew infection, there are several sprays (including apple cider vinegar and even milk sprays) that can help mitigate the effects of the mildew.

MARIJUANA PLANT CARE

MARIJUANA DISEASES – FUSARIUM

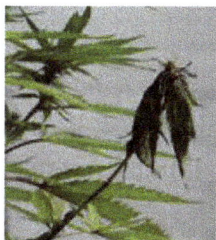

Fusarium is a fungus that lives in the soil and affects the root systems of marijuana. Obviously, hydroponic systems are not going to be susceptible to the effects of fusarium because it needs soil to survive. It most commonly produces fusarium wilt or fusarium root rot, both of which can wind up killing the plants in your marijuana garden. Fusarium can also be inactive in the soil for years only to pounce on your entire marijuana crop.

If fusarium strikes, there's really not a lot you can do in the way of treating it. It's a difficult fungus to deal with precisely because it is so difficult to spot. There are several things you can do to prevent fusarium from ever taking hold (for instance, using your own soil in containers), but if you're growing marijuana in nature, you always run the risk of fusarium being present in the soil.

MARIJUANA DISEASES – VERTICILLIUM WILT

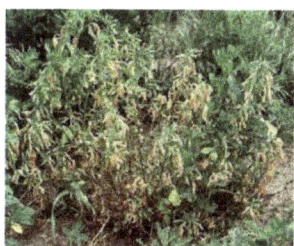

Verticilium wilt is a lot like fusarium wilt, only the former is more attracted to soils that are improperly drained or too rich. The first signs of verticilium wilt are drooping and yellowing lower leaves. The fungus will also cause the stem to turn brown at the point where it enters the soil. With these kinds of fungal diseases, it's difficult to really work around them. You really need to have a good understanding of the soil and compost mixture that you have in the ground so that you don't incur verticilium wilt.

Try to make sure that your soil drains well, so that verticilium wilt won't rear its ugly head. Because there's really no cure for verticilium wilt, it's vital that you employ good cultivation practices like crop rotation.

MARIJUANA PLANT CARE

MARIJUANA DISEASES – ROOT ROT

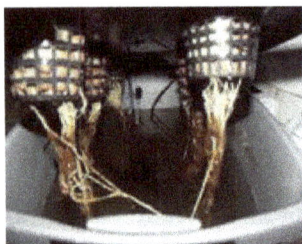

Root rot (or as it is scientifically known, pythium) is fungal disease that attacks the roots of the marijuana plant. It can appear in soil-based, container, or hydroponic growing mediums meaning that virtually no grower is safe from the power of pythium. The first sign of pythium is that the leaves will turn a brown or yellow color and the plant will start to wilt as a whole. But, if you really want to ensure that it's pythium, then you'll have to check the roots.

The roots of pythium-infected plants will start to show signs of discoloration. Eventually, the outer layer of the roots will fall off to reveal a stringy, weak inner core. Obviously, the first thing you want to do is create environmental conditions that are not conducive to the formation of root rot. Keeping your hydroponic system clean or ensuring proper drainage of a soil-based medium is important in warding off pythium.

MARIJUANA DISEASES – DAMPING OFF

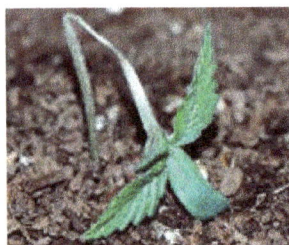

Damping off is actually a response to a disease (like pythium) rather than an actual disease itself. It is most prevalent in marijuana seedlings that have been attacked by a particular bacterium. The seedlings will start to wilt and you may just think that you're overwatering the plants, but, in reality, the roots themselves are being affected. You'll start to notice lesions in the seedling after a while before the marijuana plant just completely dies out.

It's always important to use proper preventative measures in order to avoid fungal diseases and the damping off that they produce. Seedlings won't be able to make a recovery in most instances, so preventing damping off from the start is the way to go. Making sure that the soil drains properly and underground air flow is not impeded should be your first course of action. It's the best way to ensure that spores will not take hold and you can end up with healthy, thriving marijuana plants into old age.

ENVIRONMENTAL STRESSES

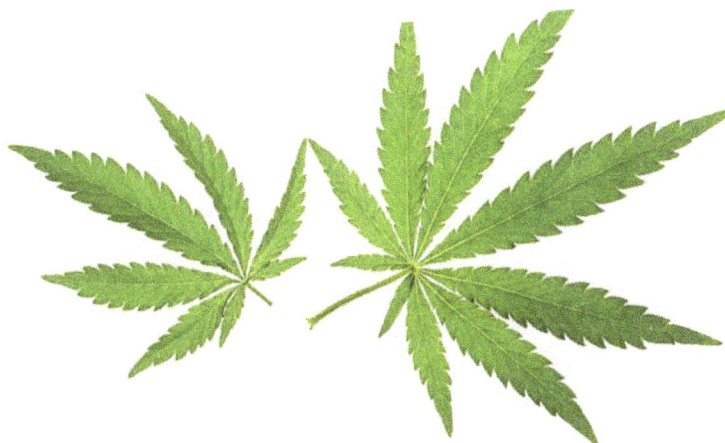

MARIJUANA PLANT CARE

EFFECT OF ENVIRONMENTAL STRESSES ON MARIJUANA PLANTS

All environmental factors work together to produce effects on your marijuana plants. Things like humidity, air quality, temperature, and light all play a role in how well or how poorly your marijuana plants will grow. Achieving ideal environmental conditions is tough work for some growers, but it can be done of you are diligent. There are some things that can affect how well the plants grow even if the rest of the environmental factors are in perfect condition.

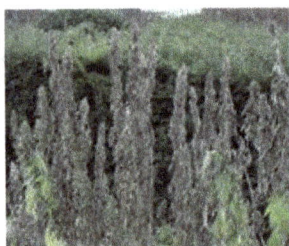

Some of these things include nutrients, the pH balance, and the length of the growing season you have allotted for yourself. Finding the right balance of both the environment and human influence is important, especially when you get your final product. Plants that grow and mature under ideal conditions will produce better weed and generally large quantities of weed as well.

DARK CYCLE INTERRUPTED – NO FLOWERS

One of the major environmental stresses that a plant can incur is changes in light intensity or dark cycle interruptions. Plants growing outdoors will get a full complement of sunlight, but indoor plants require an almost constant regimen of light. It's also true that outdoor plants have a natural, internal clock that lets them know when it's time to flower. If you're growing indoors, you can't rely on the plant's internal clock because you manipulate the amount of light that the plant receives.

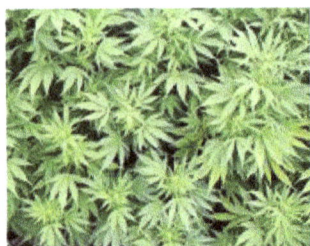

Every marijuana plant requires a certain amount of uninterrupted darkness for flowering to be induced and every strain has a different threshold for that to happen. Making sure you keep the plants in uninterrupted darkness is of the utmost importance if you want your plants to get out of vegetative state.

104

MARIJUANA PLANT CARE

HOT OR HUMID MARIJUANA GROW ROOM

Marijuana can survive under a variety of different conditions, but if the grow room is either too hot or too humid, then you can risk stressing the plants. The plants simply can't thrive if they are not provided with the right temperature and the right level of humidity. To reduce humidity, you can use a dehumidifier. This effectively replaces the moisture in the air with drier air.

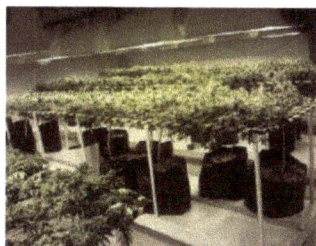

Many marijuana varieties can stand a little heat, but there's a point at which it becomes too much. Anything above the mid-80's Fahrenheit is probably too high for many varieties. You can use air conditioners to keep the room cool, or just make sure that the water is cool enough to lower the temperature of the roots.

WHEN AND HOW TO PRUNE MARIJUANA PLANTS?

Pruning can have a number of beneficial effects on the yield that a marijuana plant will provide to you. It's a common practice for farmers to prune their tomato plants to get more of a harvest when they finally mature. Marijuana works in a similar fashion. Pruning is employed by experienced growers who want to make the most of their harvest, but it is not something that should be done with too much vigor.

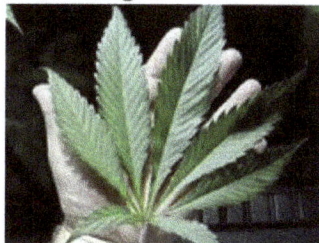

Excessive pruning can end up hurting the plant more in the long run, so it's important to prune in moderation. You can prune leaves or even buds to get more out of each marijuana plant. Pruning the top bud will produce more, small branches composed of a bounty of smaller buds. Pruning leaves allows

MARIJUANA PLANT CARE

the plant to focus all of its energy to more important growth areas (like buds). You can also prune plants for cosmetic or security purposes if need be.

AIRY AND LOOSE MARIJUANA BUDS

Loose, airy buds lack the quality of tight, firm buds both in texture and in smoke. These problems are often caused by a confluence of environmental factors including lack of light, lack of nutrient value, and/or temperatures that were too high. In most cases, high temperatures are going to be your main culprit. If you're inside, you can use air conditioners or try to move the plants as far away from the light source as possible to mitigate heat transfer. If you're outdoors, you can use a micro-sprayer system to avoid loose, airy buds.

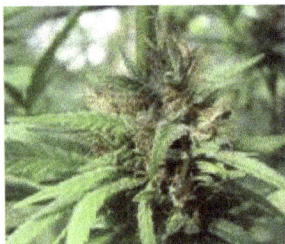

Lack of potassium during mid- to late-flowering might also be a problem, so make sure you change the fertilizer or nutrient solution to one with a higher concentration of potassium.

MARIJUANA PLANT CARE

MARIJUANA CLONES – CUTTINGS WON'T ROOT

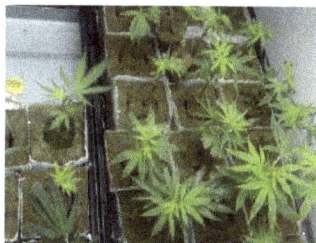

When it comes to cloning marijuana plants, your main goal should be to get the cuttings to root. Manually trying to get the cuttings to root is your best option, but there are mechanical options at your disposal as well. Sometimes the cuttings won't root in the soil that they're introduced to, but it just takes a little rooting gel and some ideal environmental conditions for the clones to take root.

You might also wonder whether it's feasible to take cuttings from marijuana plants that are mature or are flowering. The answer, of course, is yes. You can take cuttings from a plant at virtually any stage. As long as you put those clones in planting medium that supports their existence, then you should be all right. Again, maintaining a balance of humidity, temperature, and light is also important when you are trying to get <u>clones to take root</u>.

STRETCHING MARIJUANA PLANTS

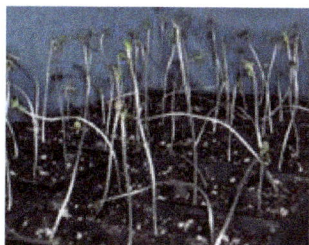

Marijuana plants that are stretched out tend to be that way because of certain environmental factors. Stretched out marijuana plants will not produce sturdy stems that can support several branches, buds, and leaves. So, it's important to ensure that the marijuana plants aren't stretching out too thin. A simple solution to this problem is to bend the stem back and forth. While this might seem to put a lot of stress on the plant, it actually forces the stem to tear and then rebuild in that space. The stems become much sturdier as a result.

Other solutions to this problem include using an excess of blue light, maintaining temperatures at around 80*F, or making sure that plants have all the light they need available to them. If light is scarce, the plants will start to elongate in order to reach the light source.

Marijuana Plant Care

LOW AND HIGH TEMPERATURE

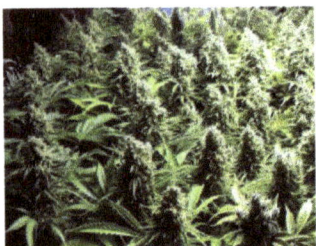

Extremes of high and low temperatures can affect marijuana plants in different ways. The ideal temperature is around 80*F, but there is some leeway in relation to this number. In fact, you can drop about 15 degrees at night if need be. Still, temperatures that are too low tend to produce plants that grow slowly and don't produce as much by harvest time. You may not notice the shift, but your yield will be much smaller than it could have been. Fixing this is really a matter of heating the grow room if it becomes too cold.

High temperatures can also cause problems with airy, elongated stalks and stems, and wilting, droopy plants overall. It's necessary to think about ventilation in this case and how it affects the temperature. You may also need to introduce air conditioning or water-cooled lights to give your grow room a break.

CAN STRESS CAUSE HERMAPHRODITE MARIJUANA PLANTS

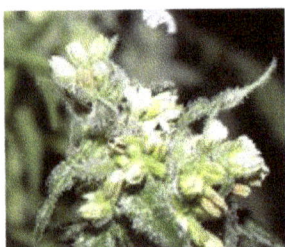

Hermaphroditism in cannabis is not ideal for growers. Many of the marijuana plants can be self-pollinating and the resultant smoke of these plants is not as good as sinsemilla buds. Stress can cause hermaphroditism in marijuana plants, but the plants may also have been genetically predestined to be hermaphroditic. It's important to avoid any major environmental changes that might induce hermaphroditism.

For instance, it's possible for plants to be growing fine in outdoor conditions, but, when you take them inside, they could be put under a lot of stress. This stress can produce hermaphroditism in those marijuana plants. The only way to deal with hermaphroditism once it exhibits itself is to try and pick off the male flowers so that the plant doesn't self-

MARIJUANA PLANT CARE

pollinate or pollinate other plants around it. You also don't want to have hermaphroditic seeds because then every subsequent generation will be composed almost exclusively of <u>hermaphroditic plants.</u>

MARIJUANA SEEDS WON'T GERMINATE

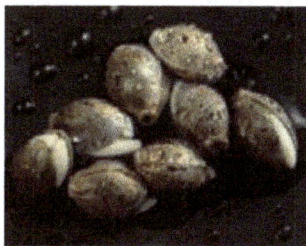

The last thing you want with your marijuana seeds is the inability to germinate. Sometimes, it's not enough to give the seed light and soil and water. In fact, it really only needs water to germinate, but other environmental factors have to work in your favor as well. The humidity, temperature, and the age of the seed itself all play a role in how effectively the seeds will germinate.

To speed up germination, you can try soaking the seeds in a hydrogen peroxide and water mixture. It can take seeds between 2 and 10 days to germinate. Outdoor seeds need to be planted at the same time of year that corn is planted in your area.

MY MARIJUANA PLANT WAS KNOCKED DOWN

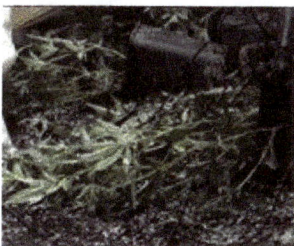

If a marijuana plant is knocked over after a storm or some particularly harsh winds, all is not necessarily lost. You need to get the marijuana plants back into position and repair any breakage that might have occurred. You also need to make sure that the plant is firmly in the ground and won't be knocked down by any subsequent storms or wind gusts. Stakes can help support a fallen over marijuana plant and tape or rope can help support cracks in the stem or stalks.

Marijuana Plant Care

Sometimes the roots are ripped out of the soil and it's necessary to cover them with a nice layer of soil. You don't want the roots to be exposed to the air for too long. Plants can occasionally be damaged so much that lifting them to an upright position is unfeasible. Still, you can salvage the plant's life my being gentle with it.

CHLORINE, SULFUR, SODIUM IN WATER – HARD OR SOFT WATER

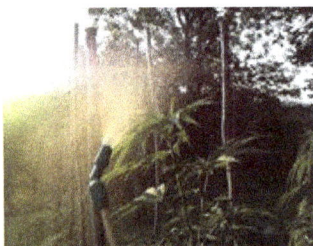

Water is one of the main ingredients in keeping your marijuana plant's healthy and thriving, but it can also be composed of some less desirable minerals. Tap water is rarely just pure H2O and it can have chlorine, sulfur, sodium, and a bevy of other minerals that can affect the growth of your marijuana plants. Hard water also introduces dissolved solids into the water, and it's important to know what your plants are receiving when you irrigate them.

There are several filters that you can buy that will get rid of the dissolved solids. Still, you don't necessarily want to use water softeners because they can end up putting too much sodium in the water. Sulfur is highly acidic can affect the nutrient uptake of the plants while chlorine doesn't appear to have a major effect on the way the plants grow.

COLD, RAINY AND HUMID WEATHER

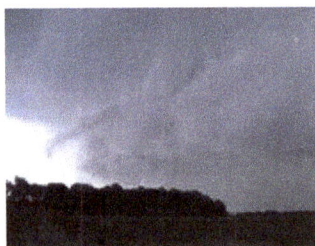

If you're growing marijuana outdoors, you're always going to have to deal with unpredictable weather patterns. Excessively cold weather obviously has a chance to ruin an entire crop because when temperatures drop below 45*F for extended periods of time, the plants stop growing. If a cold spell lasts longer than you

MARIJUANA PLANT CARE

anticipated, you may have to heat the marijuana plants artificially or even transfer them indoors.

Humid and/or rainy weather offers similar problems that you'll have to deal with. Both leave the plant susceptible to mold, and you'll want to make sure they are as dry and warm as possible after the rains have fallen or the humid weather has passed. Rain also has the chance of bringing storms that can physically affect the plant. You need to make sure that ~~~tions in mind when it comes to cold, rainy, and humid weather.

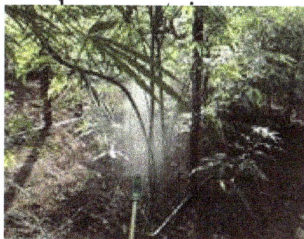

Overwatering And Underwatering Marijuana Plants

Watering your plants is a science that you'll figure out over time. You don't want to let them go without water for too long, but you also don't want to give them too much water. Depriving the plants of water produces wilting and a lack of vigor. You should never wait until the plants start to droop before you actually decide to water them. Check the moisture in the soil even if the plants look fine. If the soil is dry, then you should likely water the plants.

On the flip side, you never want the plant to be drowned by water. Too much water can produce a condition in which the plant's roots can't get enough oxygen. Make sure the soil drains properly so that it's not just collecting water around the roots and drowning them out.

Marijuana Plant Care

MARIJUANA SOIL PROBLEMS

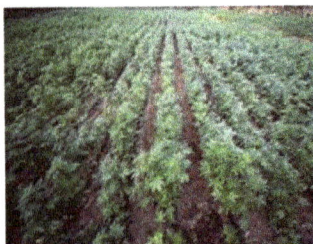

When growing marijuana outdoors, there are a number of different soil types that you will encounter. Not all soil is created equally, though, and you may wind up in an area that doesn't have good soil to work with. Clay soils, sandy soils, and dried-out soils are all types that have major detriments for growing marijuana. For instance, clay soils often don't drain well (or at all), which leaves the marijuana plants susceptible to drowning in water.

By contrast, sandy soils allow the water to go straight through them so that the plant doesn't actually get any of the nutrients. Dried-out soil is tough to work with, but, if you use a wetting agent, you can make it much more malleable.